THE CHINESE ART OF HEALING

THE CHINESE
ART
OF HEALING

Stephan Pálos

HERDER AND HERDER

3456789   BPBP   79876543
HERDER AND HERDER NEW YORK
232 Madison Avenue, New York 10016

Original edition: *Chinesische Heilkunst, Rückbesinnung auf eine grosse Tradition,* © 1963 by Dr. Stephan Pálos, Munich, Delp'sche Verlagsbuchhandlung, 1966. The title of the original Hungarian edition: *A hagyományos kinai gyógyitás.*
Translation by Translagency, Ltd.

CONTENTS

v

PART II: TRADITIONAL METHODS OF TREATMENT

FOREWORD

THIS is to my knowledge one of the first comprehensive books on Chinese medicine, written by someone thoroughly familiar with the subject, to be published in English. This subject is of particular interest at this time for two reasons. First, Chinese medicine, especially acupuncture treatment, is being used more and more in Europe by medical doctors, and even in some hospitals, as research conducted in universities and institutes is in many respects confirming its efficacy. Professional interest in Chinese medicine has recently begun to grow in the United States as well.

Secondly, the continuing discovery of undesirable side effects, some minor and others serious, of modern synthetic drugs, without denying the value of those drugs that are more than merely palliative, underlines the importance of a method of treatment that has no side effects.

With the ascendancy of China as the third world power, Chinese civilization in its various aspects has become more a focus of attention. The new China, after rediscovering during the Second World War the effectiveness of acupuncture in healing, has established medical schools in which this so-called traditional medicine is scientifically investigated, taught, and practiced in the attached hospitals. Its results are compared, and found to be superior at times, to those of Western medicine, which is also taught in the medical schools.

As a physician who has had many years of firsthand experience in the practice of Chinese medicine in addition to and in conjunction with Western medicine, I would like to attempt in these introductory remarks to dispel certain popular notions about Chinese medicine. For these notions are misconceptions arising from a lack of knowledge of the methods and practice and of the results of scientific investigation being undertaken in this field.

Acupuncture was first introduced into Western medicine in 1683, when the Dutch physician Ten Rhyne wrote a treatise on the subject. In the early nineteenth century Berlioz, physician and father of the composer, published a positive account of the results he had had with acupuncture treatment, which by that time was being used by at least some physicians. However, it was not until the middle of the twentieth century, when Soulié de Morant translated some of the basic Chinese medical texts, that acupuncture took a firmer hold in the West. Today there are medical societies for acupuncture in several countries, as well as an International Medical Society for Acupuncture, and the method is continuing to win more adherents because of its success.

Meanwhile, scientific research has begun to yield some interesting results. In 1898 the English neurologist Henry Head discovered zones on the skin, named after him, which become hypersensitive to pressure when an organ connected by nerves to this skin region is diseased. In more recent years, Russian physiologists have carried out extensive studies utilizing encephalography, electrocardiography, and X-ray. Studies involving the measurement of the electrical potential of the skin at the classical acupuncture points have verified the basic claims for acupuncture, and have related its effect to reflex action. The skin might be thought of as a screen on which the inner organs are projected through nerve connections; or as part of a telephone relay system, in which the stimulation of a certain point by a pin prick spreads through reflex action to the nerve-connected inner organ. The fundamental process of homeostasis, that is, the tendency of the organism to maintain an internal balance level, would use such stimulation as a regulating factor through which normal activity is restored.

There are about 690 acupuncture points on the skin, clustering along fourteen major lines called meridians. Experiments have shown that electrical conductivity on these points is much higher than on the rest of the skin. Since these points have anatomically determined positions, they can be located on animals. Experiments with animals have proven the interrelationship of certain skin points and inner organs. For example, a gall bladder fistula was experimentally induced in a horse by a Rumanian team of investigators, and when a point said to be related to the gall bladder was pricked, there was an increased flow of bile. This did not occur when other skin points were pricked.

Veterinarians are having success in using acupuncture in the treatment of animals. At the Veterinary Medical Institute of Alfort, under the direction of Professor Bresson, the French veterinarian Milin conducted a five-year study using cats, dogs, and horses. Animals that had not responded to the usual treatment responded to acupuncture. The success of acupuncture in the treatment of animals should dispel any notion that positive results are due to a suggestive influence of the treatment.

Besides acupuncture, traditional Chinese medicine includes a therapeutic method of breathing control and systematic breathings exercises, the *T'ai-chi-ch'üan*. As a more dynamic system of body movements than the Indian system Yoga, this therapy is receiving growing attention in the West. Further, there is an exceedingly rich pharmacopoeia which deserves more study. Empirical evidence has begun to verify in terms of the Western medical system traditional Chinese medicine's seemingly superstitious claims for the medicinal value of often utterly strange substances, such as, for example, dried lizard skin, which has been found to contain adrenalin.

Chinese thought is less causally oriented than is Western thought. It observes phenomenological correlations and perceives such correspondences as between the outer surface of the body and its inner organs. Thus it was the Chinese mind that, beginning with an accidental occurrence which has certainly been experienced by people in other parts of the world—the disappearance of pain when a point on the skin was pricked—followed up such observations and developed them into the Chinese art of healing.

William Gutman, M.D.
New York City

INTRODUCTION

THE achievements of China's ancient culture are known to everyone. Paper, porcelain, and natural silk all originated in China and were passed on from nation to nation till they spread throughout the whole world. The manufacturing processes themselves were either adopted or rediscovered by the West. China's lasting contributions to civilization are not, however, confined to astronomy, printing, or the other inventions that we have just now mentioned. A wealth of experience in the art of healing, accumulated over thousands of years, has enabled her to achieve notable results in that field as well, and their importance is gaining increasing recognition from modern medical science. The Soviet Academy of Sciences has in fact set up a special department to conduct the relevant investigations, and in France and Germany technical periodicals are devoted exclusively to the subject of acupuncture.

The aim of this book is to make the reader acquainted with the various traditional Chinese methods of healing. Although we are concerned mainly with those procedures which can stand up to scientific criticism, we also make due mention of dogmatic opinions propounded down through the course of years, together with various superstitions and the "consultation" which was once a habitual feature of the art of healing. At the same time we have tried to present scientific explanations for the various methods of treatment, although it must be admitted that the interpretations are not always conclusive or consistent. It must also be remembered that China has only recently begun to develop as a modern state, and that scientific work carried out over a period even of some decades is not enough to collate, sift, and evaluate this vast and varied wealth of cultural material. Western medical science is only now beginning to learn about many traditional Chinese methods of healing, and cannot as yet provide a complete explanation of all the processes involved. Furthermore, as far as culture is concerned, China presents a pattern of perpetual internal change, thus making it impossible for us to fill in the gaps in our knowledge and thus evaluate research findings in their final form and last detail.

Moreover, the Chinese cultural inheritance is interspersed at all levels with various philosophical influences, so that attempts are made to interpret this vast accumulation of experience by means of theses which even today cannot be entirely proved or disproved. Modern science in China is at pains to select and explain usable methods, and rejects all unscientific and superstitious non-essentials. A start was made on this work, which requires the utmost circumspection, after the end of the Revolution, using modern methods of medical science.

Under these circumstances we cannot adopt any final, positive attitude, nor is that our aim. What we propose to do is rather to make this wealth of age-old experience available and to collate such interpretations of it as have already been recognized as acceptable. Several works have indeed already been published on Chinese medical methods, the earlier ones from the point of view of general interest, but subsequent ones with the object of broadening scientific knowledge.

It is only during the last decade that any modern medical source material has become available in Chinese, so that it was thus possible for us to use such hitherto inaccessible Chinese sources, and others as well, in the writing of this book. In addition, we considered it essential to provide a short summary of both Chinese and Western technical literature on the subject of the traditional methods of healing, together with a chronological table of Chinese cultural history for ease of reference.

We also think it is worth mentioning that there are frequently very great discrepancies between the Chinese and Western sources. The Western books often quote deductions or personal opinions which may represent a revaluation rather than an interpretation of the traditional Chinese art of healing. It must also be admitted that even in the technical field such popular treatment has gained credence in certain quarters in the West, although it often does more harm than good to the credibility of Chinese medicine. Works of this kind frequently give the impression that Chinese medicine is a source of mysterious and supernatural wisdom that can no longer be comprehended by present-day medical science. From all this it might be easy to conclude that Western medicine was inadequate.

The first written documents on the subject of the Chinese art of healing date back to the 14/13th centuries B.C. Inscribed on *oracle bones* which were brought to light as the result of excavations were the characters for various diseases. The 3500 years which have passed since the appearance of the first written characters pose a great many problems, for the history of Chinese medicine also affects matters concerning archeology, early history, philosophy, and the interpretation of written texts. It is a well-known fact, for example, that Chinese writing is based on pictures which underwent a certain change in meaning with the passage of time. The meaning of the characters widened and altered frequently; some ceased to form part of normal usage, others took on a new significance. And whereas ordinary people had names for illnesses and medicaments, the written word was only comprehensible to educated persons. Those who could write often used the characters representing the colloquial words when they wanted to denote medical terms; but, in certain cases where there was no suitable character available, they often took the symbols for common, similar-sounding words as a basis, and either altered them slightly or used them in unaltered form but with a wider meaning.

The oracle bones were replaced by bamboo strips, then by pieces of material or silk, until finally the invention of paper in the 1st century B.C. and of the printed sheet in the 9th century A.D. increased the potential scope of written communication. As a result, the volume of written comment on medical works increased to such an extent that the sense of many ancient books varied according to the historical degree of development or to the religious conception. Various items were inserted into the text although they had originally nothing to do with it at all. On the other hand, such a volume of comment was useful inasmuch as it rescued for posterity works or fragments of works which we should not otherwise have known about. It is from these commentaries, often at complete variance with each other, that we learn of the bitter strife which went on between the hair-splitting, philosophizing protagonists of the various schools of thought.

There are also many medical works where in parts the sense is still not clear to the modern researcher; these texts may, in fact, perhaps have become confused centuries ago. The only way to obtain an accurate interpretation is by means of further research and a critical examination of the text.

Before dealing in detail with the various branches of the Chinese art of healing it may be pertinent to note that China comprises a vast area, and that within this area—whether divided up into small principalities or as one single state— various empirical sciences have developed according to differ ent climatic conditions and various particular natural and environmental factors. The traditions which arose and were imposed in this way were in many respects unique; in many cases, being interspersed with philosophical and religious convictions, they actually hindered development. China did not become acquainted with the modern medicine developed in the West until the First Opium War (1839–1842). Western medicine was not thought much of at first, but it later became increasingly popular as the result of many tangible successes. It became even more and more widespread after the People's Revolution of 1911 and less and less respect was paid to the native Chinese medical legacy. People failed to realize the significance of this fund of valuable experience which had been so carefully preserved through thousands of years, and no special efforts were made to save it. Only now has a start been made to rehabilitate it and to take stock of what remains. In 1954 the Government called upon doctors, with their modern training, to conduct research into the traditional Chinese art of healing and to prove and determine its intrinsic values so that they might once again serve the common good.

We have attempted in this book to summarize the results so far achieved as a result of this monumental task.

This is not a medical textbook, although we have tried to meet the experts' requirements to a considerable extent. We have sought to make the interested, educated reader acquainted with recognized principles and methods of the Chinese art of healing and also with the modern interpretation of the results it has achieved.

The book is divided into two parts. Part I states the basic principles which it is essential to grasp before the individual methods of treatment can be understood. It also describes the historical development and the intellectual trends which so strongly influenced the spread and continued development of the Chinese art of healing.

Part II describes the individual methods of treatment together with their modern interpretation. Finally, we take up the present-day place of traditional medicine in the Chinese People's Republic.

The author would like to thank the Chinese Medical Society in Peking and Professor W. G. Wogralik of Gorki for their courtesy and assistance in making Chinese and Russian material available and in supplying information on the results of the research carried out into the traditional Chinese art of healing.

PART I

GENERAL PRINCIPLES

1

A HISTORY OF THE CHINESE ART
OF HEALING

MEDICAL DOCUMENTS AND WORKS

THE legendary account by Confucius, as it has come down to
us, traces China's early history back some thousands of years
prior to the birth of Christ. Shên-nung, who invented the plough,
the Yellow Emperor, to whom dress and ceremonies are attributed, even Yü the Great, who ruled the rivers, are all
legendary figures, and the legends themselves probably arose in
the 11/13th centuries B.C., during the so-called Chou period.
North and Central Chinese archeological finds dating back to
the Neolithic Age cannot be reconciled with them. During the
second millennium B.C. the ruling family was the Shang or, as
it was later called, Yin dynasty. At the beginning of the present
century excavations in the northern part of what is now the
province of Honan brought to light valuable finds dating from
the Shang-Yin period, including characters written on bones
which were used for prophesying.[1] Here there are also to be
found, for the first time, characters referring to various diseases,
including the character for "mange."

The first written finds, however, tell us nothing of medicine;
they merely give the names of diseases and plants which were
later used for medical purposes. Thus, in the great collection of
lyrics called the *Book of Songs* (*Shih Ching*), a large part of
which was compiled in the 10/6th centuries B.C., we find the
names of a large number of plants later commonly used in
medicine, including, for example, mugwort (*artemisia vulgaris*).

3

The *Book of Changes* (*I Ching*) is of fundamental importance for the art of healing; in it are to be found fragments supposedly dating from the first half of the first millennium B.C. In the appendix, entitled "Hsi-tz'û," the terms *"Yin"* = negative (for dark, cold, feminine) and *"Yang"* = positive (for light, warm, masculine) appear for the first time. These terms originally represented the two basic opposing elements in the world, all phenomena being created by their continuous interplay. Medicine adopted this conception and—as we shall see later—altered it to suit its own ends. Thus the terms *"Yin"* and *"Yang"* not only became the starting point for future deliberations; they were also the source of misconceptions.

The second basic work is the chapter entitled "The Great Principle" (*Hung Fan*) from the *Book of Scriptures* (*Shu Ching*). In the form in which it has been handed down to us this work dates from the Han period, but it may well be that certain chapters were written as early as the first half of the first millennium B.C. It is in this chapter that mention is made for the first time of the harmony between Man and the Universe, the five elements and the division into these elements of the Universe and the world of Man. The link between North and the element of water, between South and the element of fire, between East and the element of wood, between West and the element of metal, and between Center and the elements of earth is a teaching frequently commented on in the traditional art of healing.

Historical works have likewise enabled many medical traditions to be handed down. Quite valuable, for example, is the commentary entitled *Tso Chuan,* which is said to have been compiled by Tso Chiu-ming, who lived between the 5th and 3rd centuries B.C. It contains the first mention of acupuncture. In the *Historical Records* (*Shih Chi*), written during the 1st century B.C., we find an account of the life of the celebrated doctor Pien Ch'üeh, who lived approximately about the 5th century B.C. He was the first to have made diagnoses by feeling the pulse of a patient. Similar medical contributions are found in the book entitled *History of the Late Han Dynasty* (*Hou Han Shu*), dating back to the 5th century A.D., and in many other places as well. In the course of time this medical knowledge was now and

4

then collected in large encyclopedias and lexicons, as well as in literary documents which deal with specific illnesses, give accounts of the lives of doctors, and refer to medical works. One of these is the *Encyclopedia of the Emperor Tai Tsung (T'ai-p'ing Yü Lan)*, which contains 1015 chapters. Another large collection is the *Imperial Encyclopedia (Ku-chin T'u-shu Chi-ch'êng)*, published in 1726 A.D.; it had 10,084 chapters and summarized the entire range of scientific, including medical, knowledge as it then was.

The first specifically medical work is the collection entitled *The Yellow Emperor's Classic of Internal Medicine (Huang-ti Nei-ching)*. Here Li Chu-kuo presumably collated, around the year 26 A.D., all the popular books on medicaments and the medical writings of the previous centuries. Some parts of the collection certainly date back to the 3rd century B.C., and others are possibly even older. But Li Chu-kuo did not merely collect; he also revised. The collection is in the form of a conversation; the Yellow Emperor talks most of the time with Ch'i Po, his court physician, about the relationship between Man and Nature, about the elements, and about the causes and cures for illnesses. They discuss the medical importance of *Yin-Yang*, acupuncture, and moxibustion, while massage and respiratory therapy are also mentioned. The collection was later divided into two main parts, referred to as "Su Wên" and "Ling Shu." Even modern medical literature perpetuates this division.

A similar old work is *The Book of Ailments (Nan Ching)*, attributed to the famous doctor Pien Ch'üeh, who lived in the 5th century B.C., although it may well not have originated till the Han period, in the 3rd or 2nd century B.C. According to tradition, Pien Ch'üeh was an outstanding doctor of his time, and wished to create a rational basis for medicine in the fight against superstition. It is said of him that he once examined the prince of the Kuo state, who was prostrate and unconscious, felt his pulse and ascertained that he was alive, and soon had him on his feet again with the help of various medicaments.[2]

Some time during the 2nd/3rd centuries B.C., Chang Chung-ching, or Chang Chi as he was also called, wrote two famous medical books, *Treatise on the Various Kinds of Fevers (Shang-han Lun)* and a *Short Version of the Golden Shrine (Chin Kui*

5

Yao Liieh). Both works are concerned in detail with acupuncture, moxibustion, respiratory therapy, physiotherapy, and massage. The list of medicaments includes febrifuges, diuretics, emetics, sedatives, and stimulants, and also a number of pain-killing drugs. His works are among the most significant medical books of the period.

A contemporary of Chang Chung-ching was Hua T'o, the pioneer of anaesthesia. His book has unfortunately not survived, and all we know of his life are the few details contained in the *History of the Late Han Dynasty* (from the *Hou Han-Shu Chronicles*[3]). According to his biography he began to dabble in medicine in order to help the countless soldiers wounded in the many wars. He mixed drugs with wine and used the concoction as an anaesthetic when he operated. The military despot of the period, Ts'ao Ts'ao, suffered from headaches, and the spells cast by his court magicians had no effect. Hua T'o cured him. Ts'ao Ts'ao thereupon wished to have such medical knowledge for his own use alone, and proposed making him his court physician, but the doctor declined. The despot then cast him into prison and later ordered him executed. According to another version, T'sao Ts'ao feared that the doctor sought to take his life, and for that reason had him executed. In prison, Hua T'o wrote a book on the art of healing in which he summarized his entire knowledge and experience, but he destroyed it because the prison governor was not prepared to take it into safe keeping; and thus the prescription for his anaesthetic was lost.

This outstanding doctor also composed movement exercises for strengthening the body that were based on imitations of the movements of tigers, deer, bears, apes, and birds.

A famous 3rd-century A.D. work is the *Book of the Pulse* (*Mai Ching*). The author, Wang Shu-he, lists far more methods of feeling the pulse than are known to modern medicine. The book is one of the basic works of the traditional Chinese art of healing so far as concerns the taking of the pulse. This distinguished doctor also wrote a commentary, still of importance today, on *The Yellow Emperor's Classic of Internal Medicine*.

Hand in hand with such medical books was the development of pharmacological literature. The first known collection is the *Book of Medicaments of Shên-nung* (*Shên-nung Pên-ts'ao*

6

Ching), which dates from the period between the 2nd century B.C. and the 2nd century A.D. This book lists the names of all the medicaments which were then known, together with their possible uses. The authors of later pharmacopoeia all more or less used this collection as a basis, and checked it or developed it in alchemistic fashion. Naturally, the prescriptions, more than 300 in number, do not correspond to modern pharmaceutical methods. Mercury is often prescribed, as well as sulphur in combatting skin diseases.

A large number of the listed medicaments were simply popular domestic remedies. In the course of time many of these were employed by court alchemists in their attempt to make gold or discover the "elixir of eternal life." We know that, in Europe, alchemy pointed the way for what later became scientific chemistry, and a similar development took place in China. In his work *Pao P'u-tzû,* compiled in the first half of the 4th century A.D., the Taoist doctor and alchemist Ko Hung wrote about the elixir of eternal life. The results of his experiments, to judge by present-day standards, show that he succeeded in making various chemical extracts, distilled "pharmaceutical poison," and prepared a number of compounds and mixtures. A man who was at once magician, physician, and apothecary was T'ao Hung-ching, who lived at the end of the 5th century and who, in his attempt to change mercury into gold, discovered several very worthwhile medicaments.

A famous doctor at the beginning of the T'ang period was Sun Szû-miao (581–682 A.D.), whose work, *A Thousand Ducat Prescriptions (Chi'ien Chin Fang),* is concerned with basic questions affecting the art of healing as it then was, together with the most effective prescriptions for various illnesses. This period represented great progress in the art of healing, for now the prevailing philosophical and religious doctrine, Taoism, was finding a rival in Buddhism, which was then beginning to grow in influence in China. Both religions made use of medicine in order to gain followers, and from the scientific point of view their reissue of numerous medical works at this time is of vital importance. Of particular interest are the Buddhist translations of important Indian medical works into Chinese, especially the writings of the notable Indian doctors Dscharaka and Suschruta.

7

At the beginning of the 7th century A.D. the first medical training school was set up by imperial decree, some two hundred years before the founding of the one in Salerno. According to tradition some 300 doctors are said to have studied at this school, and there were outstanding teachers who instructed in acupuncture, remedial massage, and "magic spells." The latter were introduced into the art of healing through Buddhist influence, but they never played an important part. The general art of healing concerned itself with surgery, the curing of children's ailments, moxibustion, the treatment of diseases of the eyes, nose, and ears, and dentistry.[4]

During the T'ang period there was also a monumental revision of medical books. Not only were the older medical and pharmacological books updated, but new medicaments were added until the number of standard remedies reached 844. The invention of plate printing contributed greatly to the spread of medical literature.

Increasing commercial and cultural links to the outside world during the 10th to the 14th century A.D. also had a great influence on the development of medicine. In 1027 Wang Wei-i had a human figure cast in bronze on which were marked those points on the body important for acupuncture and moxibustion. The students practiced with this bronze figure in locating such points on the body.

Liu Wan-so (1120–1180?) revised *The Yellow Emperor's Classic of Internal Medicine* and reduced the listed illnesses from approximately 1500 to 17 main types. During the revision a great many errors were also eradicated. Of the views that had accumulated in the course of a thousand years, a great many proved to be erroneous, and many illnesses appeared under different names, depending on what they were called in various parts of the vast Chinese Empire. Liu Wan-so likewise reduced the number of prescriptions from over 7000 to 371 by removing all those which were obsolete, unusable, superstitious, or downright harmful. In his opinion, the successful treatment of diseases did not necessarily require expensive medicament but, rather, effective ones.[5]

In 1578 a magisterial pharmaceutical work appeared, the *Pharmacopoeia* (*Pên-ts'ao Kang-mu*). Its author, the doctor and pharmacist Li Shih-chên (1518–1593), examined the many hundreds of important medical works that had been published up to that time, collated collections of medicaments, described 1892 different medicaments in 16 categories and 60 sub-categories, and collected some 10,000 medical prescriptions. This important work is generally considered to be the most significant pharmaceutical book of the period. It spread throughout Asia and also reached the West, and was translated into Japanese, Latin, French, Russian, English, German, and other languages. Li Shih-chên is also the author of *The Eight Special Meridians* (*Ch'i-chung Pa-mai*), in which he deals with the part played by the pulse and the "special meridians" of the body.[6] The list of medical works would not be complete without special mention of the collection entitled *The Golden Mirror of the Art of Healing* (*I-tsung Chin-chien*), which appeared in 1749. Eighty leading doctors compiled it as the result of an imperial decree, and it ranks as the most important medical collection of the Ch'ing period.

The medical and pharmaceutical works that we have mentioned are merely the most outstanding among hundreds of highly important books. Even today no complete survey has yet been made of the vast amount of commentary which followed these basic doctrinal works—their scientific evaluation will be a task for future generations. At present, 4250 traditional important medical works are available in China for research purposes.

A HISTORICAL SURVEY

If we compare, from a chronological point of view, the treasures of the Chinese art of healing and the great historical personalities of Chinese medicine with the important figures and events in the history of Western medicine, it will be seen that Pien Ch'üeh, the "father of the pulse," was probably a contemporary of the Greek physician Hippocrates (460–377 B.C.), that Hua T'o and Chang Chung-ching were contemporaries of Galen, and that the bronze figure for the study of acupuncture and moxibustion was probably cast during the same period in which Avicenna wrote his *Rules of the Art of Healing* (11th century). *The Yellow Emperor's Classic of Internal Medicine* makes clear and unequivocal reference to the circulation of the blood, which was not demonstrated in Europe for another 1500 years—by the English physician and anatomist William Harvey (1578–1657). Diagnosis by means of taking the pulse (a tradition which in China is 2500 years old), anaesthesia as early as the second century B.C., and the first use of a primitive form of vaccination all show that in many respects the Chinese art of healing was advanced over its Western counterpart. Skulls found during excavations further reveal that trepanning (cranium operations) was practiced in China thousands of years ago. But if all this is so, how does one explain the subsequent progress of modern Western medicine, and the ensuing stagnation of the traditional Chinese art of healing?

To understand this situation it is necessary to have a clear picture of social and historical developments in China.

Many people believe that the traditional Chinese art of healing is composed of some mysterious and magic knowledge which derives from a long-dead "golden era" and which far exceeds modern medicine in value. This view is not correct. Chinese medicine, as with Western medicine, was also hindered in its development. It is worth remembering that medical science in the West was able, at the beginning of modern times, to free itself from the old scholastic attitude of merely observing phenomena and to introduce experiment and analytical method and thus provide its scientific theories with a basis which corresponded to practical experience. Although experiments were carried out in a methodical way and were important even at an early date mainly among alchemists, they were applied in primitive form and not consciously so, with the consequence that medical knowledge tended rather to be accumulative and synthetic. Most of it consisted of concrete experience gained originally from specific cases, and was therefore empiric. Generalization in the absence of analytical experiment could thus lead to false conclusions.[7]

Our knowledge of Chinese antiquity is mainly derived from legends and—as far as concrete evidence is concerned—from the excavations which were started around the turn of the century. The relics which have come to light, such as utensils and oracle bones, point to an archaic form of society which had not yet attained statehood and in which the *"Wang,"* that is to say, the king, had the rights and duties of a tribal chieftain. As far as the economy was concerned, animal husbandry and the tilling of the soil were quite important, but in the neighborhood of the royal palace there was a highly developed and flourishing handicrafts industry which mainly served religious worship and the strengthening of royal power. Land and slaves were public property, trade had not yet developed, and the capital city basically meant the place where the peasants had to pay their taxes. This was the peculiar patriarchal order of things which developed during the Shang-Yin period and which was also to characterize the Chou period during the first millennium B.C.

During this time the art of healing was still based on a collection of popular experience to which various elements were added. This wealth of practical experience was directed towards ensuring the health of the tribesmen, serfs, and peasants, but above all that of the king himself. Magic, of course, also had its due part to play, since often there was no natural explanation for the occurrence of an illness.

The first healers or medicine-men were a type of shaman who understood more about the healing of injuries and skin diseases than they did about the treatment of internal ailments. They also used magic spells, in which the rational and mystical elements became confused. As we have already noted, the evidence of the oracle bones suggests that the main body of knowledge at the beginning of the antique period concerned traumatic abdominal injuries, diseases of the ears, nose, eyes, mouth, and teeth, and bone fractures. Stone needles were used for opening boils and abscesses, and the principle of trepanning was also understood.

Society during the Chou period (11th–3rd century B.C.), of a patriarchal-bureaucratic kind, represented the transition from primitive culture to the antique type of state. The history of this entire epoch consists of wars fought continuously by the various principalities anxious to achieve supremacy. The land and those who tilled it remained "public property." The king personified society. It was probably at this time that the "doctrine of the

11

five elements," as described in the chapter "The Great Principle" in the *Book of Scriptures,* and the *Yin-Yang principle,* as explained in the appendix ("Hsi-tz'û") to the *I Ching,* were incorporated in the traditional art of healing.

The philosopher of the Chou period who exerted the greatest influence was K'ung-tzû, the Latinized version of whose name is Confucius; according to tradition he lived from 551 to 479 B.C. He himself did not commit his teachings to paper, but his students compiled, among other books, the work in dialogue form entitled *Discussions and Conversations (Lun-yü),* which formed an important basis for social order both at that time and subsequently. Confucius adhered basically to those moral standards which, if they are adhered to, enable a country to be governed peacefully.

The standards of Confucius ensure loyalty to the bonds of patriarchy and kinsmanship which unite the living and the dead It was also a form of loyalty towards one's ancestors that the body which one had received from one's parents should not be mutilated but be returned to one's ancestors after death in a state of completeness. This is the main reason for the primitive state of medical knowledge concerning surgery, midwifery, and anatomy. In China, amputated parts of the body were buried with the person to whom they belonged—if, indeed, the doctors went so far as to amputate at all; bodies were dissected, but— as in medieval Europe—secretly, using the corpses of hanged criminals. These traditions persisted until the Chinese Revolution, and are mentioned in both old and new literature as well as in travel accounts.

During this period there grew up, in addition to Confucianism, another philosophy which had originated among the peasantry and exerted a strong influence. It subsequently came to rival the teachings of Confucius in many parts of the country and later became known as Taoism. This philosophy is manifested in the philosophical poem entitled *Lao-tzû* or, as it was later called, *Tao-tê Ching,* ascribed to a sage known as the Lao Tan or Lao-tzû ("Old Master"). In this poem the concept and principle of the *Tao* ("Way") are described as a natural law applicable to all, in contrast to the patriarchal order of things propounded by Confucius. This philosophical movement also had a great effect

12

on the traditional art of healing, although the latter, having once abandoned its original attitude of merely observing phenomena, subsequently came to form the basis of diametrically opposed speculation, including Taoist alchemy.

In the pre-Christian epochs other methods of healing were preferred at various times in different parts of China. In the eastern sector, for example, in the area of the modern province of Shantung, treatment was carried out mainly by means of stone needles; in the western part, in the modern province of Shensi, with medicinal herbs; in the north, in the modern province of Hopei, by moxibustion; in the south, in the modern province of Hupei, with metal needles; and in central China, in the modern province of Honan, with massage.[8] The Confucians condemned all magical, faith-healing methods. Pien Ch'üeh developed the technique of pulse-taking, and philosophical teachings also gained a foothold in the art of healing.

The patriarchal aristocracy gradually found a dangerous enemy in the patrician citizens of the towns, for the latter had grown rich and aspired to power. It was they who supported Ch'in Shih Huang-ti, who united the principalities in the year 221 B.C. and who had the Confucian books burned in the year 213 in order to deprive the patriarchal aristocracy of power. The books on medicine and agriculture were, however, spared destruction, as were those on soothsaying.

The Ch'in dynasty was doomed to fall, as neither culture nor the production of goods in the towns had developed sufficiently to maintain power. The Han dynasty which followed (206 B.C.– 220 A.D.) nevertheless was able to reëstablish the patriarchal aristocracy and also maintained the unity of China. Chang Chung-ching and also Hua T'o, who was the first to use anaesthesia, lived during this period.

The transition to the Middle Ages in China was marked, as in Europe, by penetration and conquest on the part of nomadic tribes. An important turning point in the spiritual life of this epoch was the spread of Buddhism, and the same period saw translations of important medical works from various Indian languages.

The T'ang dynasty (618–907 A.D.) was a period during which both commerce and culture flourished. Although the state was

13

based on a patriarchal system of government, the feudal land-owners also had privileges, which meant that their class now had increased power vis-à-vis the emperor. The latter sought to force them back into the patriarchal framework by means of decrees and thus strengthen the power of centralized government, the maintenance of which led to a considerable development in trade and culture in the towns. The invention of plate-printing, as we have seen, also enabled medical works to become widespread. Another cultural achievement in the towns was the building of state-subsidized hospitals for the poor and lepers. The peasants, however, were hard-pressed, and the only officials whose position was secure were those who supported centralized government.

Such mounting social contrasts persisted into the Sung dynasty (960–1276 A.D.). Factories and nationwide trade developed in the towns, and institutions similar to modern banks were founded. The invention of the compass encouraged navigation and Chinese merchants were thus able to capture part of the south-seas trade carried on by the Arabs. Bank notes, too, were introduced; these were originally printed on perfumed silk. Large collected works and encyclopedias were published. A bitter struggle broke out among the doctors, however, over various changes that were being made in the old, inherited art of healing. The revival of philosophy, too, had its effect on the development of medical theory.

Neo-Confucian literature derives basic, materialistically tinted principles of Nature from the *Yin-Yang* doctrine, and attributes to the reciprocal action of these natural principles the emergence of the five elements (earth, fire, water, metal, and wood), on which all creation is based. These ideas were expressed by the philosopher Chou-tzû (or Chou Tun-i) (1017–1073 A.D.). Another contemporary philosopher, Chang Tsai (1020–1077 A.D.), maintained that the beginning and end of all things is due to the struggle between the opposing forces of *Yin* and *Yang,* and that all movement originates from this conflicting pair of opposites.

The Mongol invasion and the founding of the Yüan dynasty (1280–1368 A.D.) led to a period of terrible oppression for China. The Mongolian leaders opposed Confucianism, and as

14

a result a great deal of popular literature and medical knowledge which had hitherto been suppressed now came to light.

During the Ming period (1368–1644), after the Mongols had been driven out, there was a great upsurge in trade, which in turn strengthened the power of the towns.

Towards the end of the Ming dynasty, Europe was entering the age of discoveries. European navigators brought back spices and drugs, and so it was that camphor arrived from China together with opium, which was originally used in that country merely as a medicant.

In the 16th century, European trading companies established themselves in China; in 1516 Portuguese ships anchored off Canton. China attempted to cut herself off by refusing to allow foreigners to enter her harbors.

During this period more than 50 medical works were published in China on the subject of smallpox, and about the middle of the 16th century it was discovered that the secretion from smallpox vesicles or dried smallpox vesicles themselves in powdered form were a powerful means of immunization. The powder made from the smallpox vesicles was sniffed into the nose. This method of immunization, which moreover had long been in use in popular medicine, was also adopted by Russian doctors, who transmitted it to Turkey. As far as the West was concerned, it was not until 1717 that immunization against smallpox was discovered by an Englishman, Edward Jenner.

The great doctor and pharmacist of the Ming period, Li Shih-chên, compiled his vast *Pharmacopoeia* towards the end of this epoch. But pedantic hair-splitting and an excess of philosophical dogma prevented any real progress being made in the art of healing. Medical doctrine, overloaded with commentaries written on the commentaries themselves, reached its peak during the Ch'ing period (1644–1911), and revealed at the same time the stagnation into which China had sunk.

In 1644 the Chinese feudal lords summoned the Manchus into the country to put down the great peasants' revolt of Li Tsê-chêng; but the Manchus seized power throughout all China and founded a new dynasty (1644–1911), called the Ch'ing. They oppressed the Chinese people with all the means at their disposal, but this ruling caste feared foreign influence and therefore broke off all cultural and commercial links with neighboring countries in order to secure their power. During the reign of the emperor K'ang-Hsi (1662–1723), many astronomers were banished because they had concerned themselves with Western astronomy. Also withdrawn was the book on anatomy which the missionary Dominique Parrenin had compiled and translated into the Manchu language. The Manchu rulers preferred the Chinese to occupy themselves with producing commentaries on the classical works. Thus a period of rule by foreign emperors (nearly 270 years long) suppressed Chinese medicine largely into hair-splitting study and criticism of texts. Perhaps the only positive result of such work was the discovery that certain medical works were found to be imitations, and thus their true age was revealed.

After the First Opium War (1839–1842), the Western colonial powers secured a foothold in China, and thus hastened the dissolution of a social order which had persisted in that country for thousands of years.

After the Opium War the East India Company established hospitals in Canton and Macao. China thus became acquainted with European medicine, which aroused increased interest mainly after the introduction of anaesthesia (1846) and the use of antiseptic procedures (1867). Initially, however, there was a distrust of Western medicine, perhaps because it reached China after the defeat of the Opium War.

The centuries-long oppression under the Manchu dynasty was ended by the Revolution of 1911. Sun Yat-sên was named President of the newly constituted Republic, but from 1920 onwards there were more revolutionary struggles and civil wars, with the Kuomintang party finally emerging as victor in 1927, and Chiang Kai-shek the National President.

The Kuomintang party thought little of the heritage of traditional medicine and branded it as unscientific quackery. Chiang Kai-shek, in fact, proposed publishing a decree prohibiting those doctors from practicing who remained faithful to the traditional arts of healing; but this suggestion was met with such strong protest from the then capital, Nanking, that the government finally backed down. Nevertheless, it did do all it could to

16

restrict the activities of those doctors who observed the traditional arts, and deepened the division between those doctors who had modern training and those of the old school.

The year 1949 brought an end to the confusion and strife of civil war with the victory of the Communist Party. The first National Hygiene Conference (1950) established a new set of medical principles, one which took account of the traditional arts of healing. The Chinese People's Republic has thus called upon scientifically trained Chinese doctors to examine traditional healing according to the methods of modern science. At the same time, it has encouraged those doctors who have been trained in the traditional arts of healing to study modern medical methods. This appeal has already had significant results, which we shall later discuss.

THE INTERRELATION OF MEDICINE
AND PHILOSOPHY

In any history of medicine, some notice should obviously be given to the philosophical and social context in which it developed.

China is a vast territory with special climatic and geological features. Various therapeutic problems are endemic to particular regions. In southern China, the warmer climate zone, the types of illnesses are materially different from those of the more temperate climate conditions in the north; and those in western China differ again from those in the east, which is closer to the sea. The history of the art of healing, too, shows that different types of empirical medicine evolved in the various sectors, each adapted to local climatic conditions and each employing distinct methods. It should be remembered that, until the coronation of the first emperor (221 B.C.), the "celestial empire" of China was comprised of small and often warring principalities, and in this light one can more easily understand why the medical traditions which have come down to posterity seem confused and at variance from region to region. The written documents of South China, a politically more important and historically older region, are better preserved than those of the peripheral and more backward mountainous and desert areas of the country. These geographical differences are made even more complicated by the linguistic situation, for diseases were known by different names in different Chinese provinces. This caused a number of terminological difficulties which persist to this day.

In a consideration of the history of the Chinese art of healing from the philosophical point of view, we can differentiate five separate epochs:

  1. the epoch of simple empiricism
  2. the epoch of the formulation of theories
  3. the epoch of the development of experience and theories
  4. the epoch of divergence between theory and practice
  5. the epoch of reconstruction and synthesis.

1. The Epoch of Simple Empiricism

This era marks the beginnings of the art of healing in China. The simple observation of Nature, regard for the climatic conditions, and above all a recognition of the external symptoms of illness, all testify to a versatile, naïve empiricism accompanied by a complete lack of systemization. Observance is *ad hoc* in character and interpreted with the aid of magic elements, such as we find in the history of medicine in other cultures. During this time stone needles were used as operating instruments, and a large number of medical herbs were also employed, as was trepanning.

Since time immemorial men have crossed and re-crossed China, trading, working, or waging war. Thus items of medical knowledge travelled from one region to another, taking on lesser or more importance depending on climate and other variables.

It should be noted that the legends which tell of these early times are generally of later origin. They mostly arose once the dynasties had become settled and there was need to support their power with a hereditary sovereign title. The older medical legends and traditions, together with the reports of the deeds

18

of the legendary Shên-nung, are of later origin and thus far have not been substantiated by any relics which have come to light as a result of excavations.

2. The Epoch of the Formulation of Theories

It is not possible to give a precise date as to when this era began; all that can be definitely said is that straightforward medical empiricism only began to form a compact, uniform system once the principle of *Yin-Yang* and the "doctrine of the five elements" had provided a basis for it. From the appearance of some parts of the *I Ching* and the *Shu Ching* the era may be roughly placed in the first half of the first millennium B.C. As we shall see, the concepts of both these works were closely interwoven with medical knowledge and traditions and provided a theoretical basis for the traditional art of healing.

In addition to these doctrines the concept of the "Way" (*Tao*) as expressed by Taoism or the *Tao-tê Ching* exerted a strong influence on medical thought, since, by virtue of its particular character vis-à-vis Confucianism, it provided a splendid basis for regarding illness and good health as a phenomenon affecting all people indiscriminately and not conditionally depending on social position.

Taoism was closely linked both to the courtly life of the ruling classes and no less to the simple life of the common people. It is difficult to separate monastic and secular arts of healing in China. The way of life of the Taoist hermit-physicians was just as closely bound up with the common people as it was with life at court. What we do know is that some of the Taoist hermits led a life of meditation or occupied themselves with the cultivation of the sciences. Another group of Taoists was concerned with magic, wizardry, the conquest of the ego ("transsubstantiation"), alchemy, and matters affecting the prolongation of life. All of these elements are to be found in *The Yellow Emperor's Classic of Internal Medicine,* in which Li Chu-kuo combined and systematized all the writings and fragments concerning the art of healing from the centuries prior to the birth of Christ.

19

3. The Epoch of the Development of Experience and Theories

This period is closely associated with the beginnings and development of relationships between China and India. Contacts arose mainly as a result of Buddhist intervention. We already know from our brief historical survey that China was acquainted with Buddhism as early as the 1st century A.D., but that we cannot assume that there were any close links until the 6th century onwards. Buddhism has no caste system or any other social differences. From the various Indian philosophers it has taken over everything that offered universal knowledge instead of individual facts, giving preference to the concrete over the abstract. In addition to knowledge regarding the causes of illness and the doctrine of the "noble eightfold path," the monks also brought Indian cultural values to China and thus made known the common methods of healing applied in India. The translation of the writings of the famous Indian physicians Dscharaka and Suschruta is, as we have seen, together with that of other medical works, also due to Buddhist monks. There is one obvious reason why the monks concerned themselves with the art of healing; relief of suffering and universal kindness to all living things are fundamental principles of the Buddhist doctrine. That is why so many Buddhist monks, who were also famous doctors, feature in the history of Chinese medicine. It is because of their influence—for psychological reasons if for no other—that Chinese medicine has become of more immediate relevance to people, whereas the followers of Confucianism, and to an even greater extent those of Taoism, approached medicine from the theoretical point of view. This view is supported by the fact that the Buddhist medical descriptions which have come down to us are, despite their odd terminology, more easily understood and are more approximate to reality than the Taoist medical writings.

This exchange extended not only to practical procedures but also absorbed the way of thought of Indian philosophy. This led in China to an admixture with theoretical principles already in existence. For example, in the field of respiratory therapy there

20

are yogic elements both in Buddhism and in Chinese medicine. The spread of Buddhism in China was thus of particular importance for the art of healing, for it enriched the knowledge which had hitherto been gained both on a theoretical and practical plane and led to further development.

From the Confucian point of view, of course, the application of the surgical methods used in India was not possible, since, we have seen, Confucianism was strongly opposed on philosophical grounds to any "mutilation" of the body. This was a severe loss to the traditional Chinese art of healing, since it prevented the development of practical anatomical knowledge and surgical methods.

4. The Epoch of Divergence Between Theory and Practice

This period coincides with that of the Ming and Ch'ing dynasties and proves how closely social and philosophical history were interrelated. Until now we have spoken only of collaboration between monastic and secular medicine; now we must also discuss the opposing views of official medicine and "folk doctors." The Ming era was a time of stagnation in Chinese development, while the Ch'ing period marked its absolute nadir.

In the field of medicine at this time, commentaries on medical literature predominated over original works, and the official doctors steadily gained in influence. The grading of medical posts merely represented stages in the social hierarchy and did not equate with any corresponding degree of ability. The official state examination required basically a knowledge of such traditional works as were considered to be the classics, together with their commentaries and the various references to medicine in historical and literary works; even the writing of poems was part of the examination. Such state examinations were expensive, since they were the means of achieving social position, titles, and high office. The subtle discussions on theory resembled the threshing of empty straw more than anything else. The theoretical structure of the art of healing lost whatever little real foundation it originally had.

The official doctors rarely practiced themselves, and when they did it was only to treat a personage occupying a high social position. The common people were looked after by the so-called "folk doctors." Many of these doctors had not passed the state examination and, since they could not as a result obtain a well-endowed position, were forced to earn their living by treating the poorer classes. There were also, however, many doctors who were seriously interested in their patients and consequently did not bother with the theories of the official doctors; instead, they investigated the causes of illnesses and set down their findings in writing. As a result, important dynasties of physcians were founded, composed of doctors who had no ambition to attain official status but who followed their family tradition and devoted their efforts to the practical application of their knowledge. These doctors treated the ordinary people, who turned to them with understandable trust. The truly destitute, however, were left to treat themselves according to the scraps of knowledge which they had happened to pick up. Now and again (for they were not always communicative) what folk doctors practiced and advised was in sharp contrast to the fashionable theories held in official circles, and thus the spread of their opinions was eventually regarded as harmful to the social prestige and power of the official doctors.

Thus arose the "family traditions" and the handing down of medical knowledge from generation to generation by word of mouth to an extent unknown in the history of medicine in any other culture. Strict secrecy was the only defense against the official doctors.

Such traditional knowledge is still met with today, and is currently being collected throughout China. Compared with the purely theoretical, these "family secrets" have true medical value, since they derive from practical experience and deal mainly with the treatment of certain illnesses and complaints. Knowledge of this kind is a mine of information for research into the traditional art of healing.

5. The Epoch of Reconstruction and Synthesis

This era began with the end of the Revolutionary War (1949) and is still developing. The task of modern medical research consists of, among other things, collecting, publishing, and examining the traditional arts of healing according to scientific method.

2

MAN AND NATURE

OLD Chinese philosophy regarded the human organism as a miniature version of the universe. This is a view shared by many peoples of antiquity. Philo of Alexandria, for example, a contemporary of Seneca, was the first to refer to a man as "a small world." According to the Chinese concept, the processes which occur within the human organism—including illnesses—are connected with the interplay of the five creative elements. Man cannot therefore be divorced from Nature; he forms an organic part of it and is closely linked to the universe.[9] Thus Nature, as a macrocosm, and man, as a microcosm, obey the same laws.

The world of imagination in antique China was not bereft of analogies; the head was associated with the firmament, the hair with the stars and constellations, and the eyes and ears with the sun and the moon. Human breath, the soul, corresponded to the wind (see the Greek word "pneuma"), blood was equated with rain, while the blood-vessel system and the "humors" were the streams and rivers, and the openings in the body were the valleys, and so on. The remaining equations were also note-worthy: in the microcosm the human body is the earth itself, the skeleton represents the mountains, the heart the constellation of the Great Bear, while the five elements (wood, fire, earth, metal, and water) corresponded to the five interior organs: the lungs, heart, kidneys, spleen, and liver. The four seasons corresponded to the four limbs, the twelve months to the twelve large "sections" of the body, and the 360 days (the Chinese lunar calendar has 360 days) to the 360 small "sections" of the body.[10]

This primitive, cosmic-magical view is also reflected in the *I Ching,* in which the sky corresponds to the head and the earth to the stomach. Wang Kui († 1390 A.D.) notes in his book *Li Hai Chi* that the human body is an imitation of heaven and earth in every detail. Just as in the cyclic signs of the firmament the Virgin, the Balance, and the Archer are situated forward and above, so too are the corresponding organs, heart and lungs, situated in the upper part of the body. And just as the signs of the zodiac, Fishes, Ram, Twins, and Crab, are situated behind and below, so too are the kidneys and liver situated down below and at the rear of the human body.[11]

Similar interpretation was devised during the period of scholasticism in Europe. Among philosophical systems with like concepts is a book by Agrippa de Nettesheim (1485–1535) entitled *De occulta philosophia,* according to which the planets correspond to the Hebrew lettters of the name of Yahweh (in Hebrew, Jahve). The book also offers detailed comparisons with the nomenclature and classification of the seven angels, seven birds, seven kinds of fish, seven kinds of metal, seven kinds of stone, parts of the body, orifices in the head and the seven places of the damned.[12]

There was also in China a school of thought which compared the human body to the state. This view is to be found in the chapter entitled "Su Wên" in *The Yellow Emperor's Classic of Internal Medicine,*[13] as well as in the writings of the Taoist doctor Ko Hung, who lived in the first half of the 4th century A.D. In his book entitled *Pao P'u-tzû* he compares the thorax and the abdominal region to palaces and courts, the limbs to the frontiers, the bones and joints to the various classes of officials, the spirit to the ruler, the blood to the ministers, but energy, which keeps the whole body alive, to the people. The fact that this concept—if not in the medical sense—had a basic truth and sociological meaning becomes evident from the final conclusion: "The people provide life. If the people are fed, the state can endure; if not, then the state, too, perishes."[14]

Later Chinese thought did not continue such a primitive view.

We have mentioned it merely in order to give an overall view of the various concepts which arose in Chinese antiquity.

The empirical observations of subsequent times were based on the correct realization of the interrelationship between man and Nature. They no longer relied on magic but increased that abundance of practical knowledge which often enabled the traditional art of healing to achieve so many surprising successes. Man must therefore obey the laws of the universe, for, as a microcosm, he is an organic part of the macrocosm.

THE PRINCIPLE OF YIN AND YANG

According to the doctrine of the art of healing in Chinese antiquity, there is a constant struggle in the human organism, just as in Nature, its environment, between opposing and unifying forces. Good or bad health is determined by the fluctuations of these conflicting forces. The two polar forces in which universal energy manifests itself are known as *Yin* and *Yang*.

We have already noted that these two terms appeared for the first time in the appendix ("Hsi-tz'û") to the *I Ching*. Originally *Yin* signified the northern and *Yang* the southern side of a mountain on which the sun shone. *Yin* terms included negation, cold, dark, and female, whereas *Yang* personified positive, male, light, and warmth. Just as these two forces are in constant conflict in the universe and yet at the same time form a whole, so too do they symbolize harmony or disharmony in the human organism. An evenly balanced, equipoised *Yin* and *Yang* means good health—but if the energy is displaced in any one direction it denotes illness. Over-powerful *Yang* symbolizes increased organic activity; if, on the other hand, *Yin* predominates, this implies hypofunction. Just as the continuous interplay of these two opposing forces produces all phenomena in the universe— as, for example, the changing seasons and the sequence of night and day—so too does it produce in the human organism the inhalation and exhalation of air and the conditions of walking and sleeping. The *Yin-Yang* principle also accounts for parallels between sympathetic and parasympathetic nervous systems.

According to the "Su Wên," *Yin* and *Yang* represent the law

26

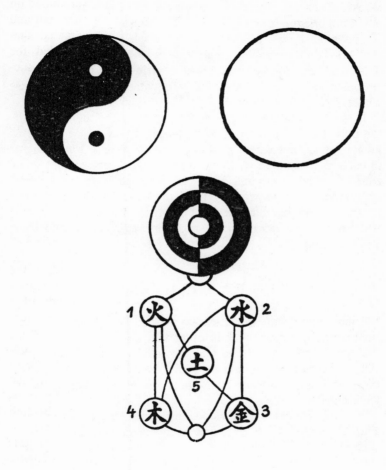

FIGURE I
YIN-YANG SYMBOLS

The figure at top left shows the old fish-shaped representation. The figure at top right symbolizes the great unity, the "limited infinity," which is the basis of all existence and the preserving principle of all living things; at the same time, however, it also represents the "great nothingness." The lower figure, an old Taoist drawing, depicts the connections between the *Yin-Yang* and the *five elements*. The individual symbols denote: 1. fire, 2. water, 3. metal, 4. wood, 5. earth.

of heaven and earth: master of all living things, mother of change, the origin of birth and death.[15] The corollary is that each illness affects the whole body, since good health represents a condition of equilibrium in the whole organism.

The official view of the Chinese People's Republic is that the *Yin-Yang* principle "contains an original, spontaneously dialectical, and simple materialistic doctrine; it is free of superstition; it approximates scientific formulation; and it represents a progressive way of thinking."[16]

Different variations of *Yin* and *Yang* are to be found both in the universe and in the human organism. Every *Yin* contains a greater or lesser element of *Yang,* and there is a *Yin* element in each manifestation of *Yang.* As we shall later see, this doctrine has allotted *Yin* and *Yang* forms of energy to the various organs according to whether the latter have passive or active functions, and has classified the internal organs according to whether they are powerful, average, or weak manifestations of *Yin* and *Yang.*

THE FIVE ELEMENTS

We shall now devote our attention at some length to the "doctrine of the five elements," in order that we may become more fully acquainted with basic Chinese medical terminology. The chapter entitled "The Great Principle" in the *Book of Scriptures* traces the harmony between Man and Universe back to these five elements.

The five elements are: wood, fire, earth, metal, and water. They can exist in a helpful and complementary relationship to each other or they can work against one another and so destroy themselves. The doctrine of the elements no doubt has its origins in very ancient concepts. It is perhaps possible to read into it such a context as: Fire is fed by wood; after the fire has burned itself out there remain ashes which become earth, in which metals are found and from which water springs; the water feeds the trees, thus completing the circle back to the element of wood.

28

Such a sequence is, in part, supported by the traditional art of healing. But in another respect the elements are in opposition to one another: the antipole of fire is metal; the antipole of earth is water. Metal and wood cancel each other out, as do water and fire, or wood and earth. The following diagram will help to make this clear.

According to the chapter headed "Hung Fan," the sequence of elements is: water, fire, wood, metal, earth. The number five,

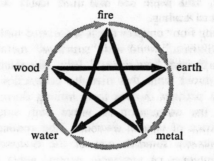

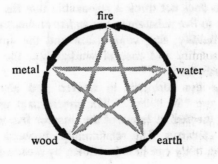

FIGURE 2
THE RELATIONSHIP OF THE FIVE ELEMENTS
The black arrows denote the directions in which the five elements "destroy" one another; the gray arrows denote the directions in which they "help" each other.

according to the same chapter, does not merely refer to the five elements but also to other groups of five, such as the five qualities of taste, the five seasons, and the five possibilities of happiness. Traditional teaching also established links between the components of the various groups, and there thus arose a closed, self-contained system; the continuous efforts to improve and refine it led the Chinese art of healing to adopt an exaggerated formalism. At the same time, numerous successful processes on a practical plane were linked to the doctrine of the five elements, and these are still used today as part of the traditional art of healing.

In the "Hung Fan" chapter fire is associated with "bitterness," water with "saltiness," wood with "sourness," metal with "sharpness," and earth with "sweetness." John Needham, the English naturalist, deduced from this that the connection between fire and bitterness perhaps derives from boiling down of medicinal herbs, while the association of water with saltiness testified to the experience of coastal dwellers. The connection between wood and sourness reminds one of the discovery of certain acidulous substances of vegetable origin, while that between metal and sharpness or pungency recalls the pungent smoke produced when metal is being melted. The association of earth with sweetness suggests wild honey or the sweet taste of corn.[17] Needham also does not think it impossible that the five elements may not refer to five substances but to five characteristics: water, representing fluidity; fire, combustion and the development of heat; wood, solidity and ease of workability; the metals, fusibility; and earth, fertility.[18]

"There are five elements in heaven and also on earth," according to the "Su Wên."[19] The macrocosm as well as the microcosm is divided in terms of the number five in accordance with the five elements. The relationships between the universe and the human body can best be shown by means of the following table:

Five elements	Five seasons	Five taste qualities	Five colors	Five atmospheric influences	Five stages of development
wood	spring	sour	blue	wind	birth
fire	summer	bitter	red	heat	growth
earth	late summer	sweet	yellow	humidity	change (puberty)
metal	autumn	sharp	white	drought	maturity
water	winter	salty	black	cold	storage

When we add to this table the five points of the compass: north, south, east, west, and center (in China the center is also a point of the compass), together with the five well-known planets: Mercury, Venus, Mars, Jupiter, and Saturn, then we have the manifestations of the five elements in Nature.

DIVISION IN TERMS OF THE MICROCOSM[21]

Five elements	Five sense organs	Five structural elements	Five Fu's	Five Tsang's	Five emotions
wood	eye	sinews	bile	liver	anger
fire	tongue	blood vessels	small intestine	heart	joy
earth	mouth	muscles	stomach	spleen	anxiety
metal	nose	hair	large intestine	lung	sadness
water	ears	bones	urinary bladder	kidneys	fear

The five *Fu's* listed in the above table refer to the active, operational inner organs, while the *Tsang's* denote the passive, storage ones.

The *Yin-Yang* principle and the five elements are closely associated. The *Yang* energy can be strengthened, but also weakened by the five elements, and the same applies to the Yin. The art of healing, too, differentiates between *Yin* and *Yang* organs; a *Yin* and a *Yang* organ belong, as we shall see later, to each element. Thus Man fits into the totality of Nature, becomes an organic

31

part of it, and thereby fulfills the *"Tao,"* the universal law of Nature.

For the sake of completeness we should also note that the *Yin-Yang* principle and the five elements are also associated with the times of day and the cyclic signs of the Chinese lunar calendar, as a result of which a connection was assumed between illness and cosmic forces. This led on the one hand to important results, for even nowadays modern biometeorology and cosmobiology are concerned with similar problems. On the other hand, such acceptance of a relation between health and illness and the position of the stars degenerated into extremes of superstition, the pressure of which affected all aspects of life—the timing of enterprises and weddings, and also the treatment of illnesses. An astrological representation of this kind is shown in Figure 3.

Thus far we have shown how the human body forms a small world comparable to the large one. This led to a kind of "philosophical anatomy," according to which Nature and the human body coincide in numerous respects. Both Nature and Man are subordinated to the *Yin-Yang* principle and the five elements.

In the medical section of this book we shall show that such a philosophical view led in certain cases to positive practical results, albeit not because of speculative altruism, but due to its empirical core. The present official policy on health matters of the Chinese People's Republic is obviously aimed at upgrading the importance attached to the traditional methods of healing. As part of this rehabilitation, as we have seen, an attempt is being made to achieve a synthesis between traditional views and prevailing political-sociological doctrine. Yet practical considerations may well play a considerable part in all this, quite apart from the impetus given by national self-assertion, for although there are some 500,000 doctors in the People's Republic of China who have been schooled in the traditional manner, there are only approximately 70,000 who have received any kind of scientific training.

To gain a fuller perspective on the modern medical situation in China, we shall now quote from a number of works recently published in the Chinese mainland and in the Soviet Union apropos the traditional art of healing.

A book entitled *Summary of the Traditional Chinese Art of*

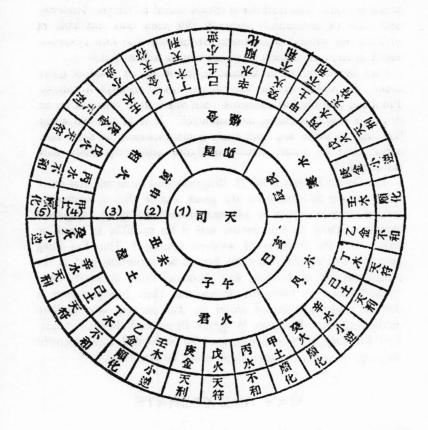

FIGURE 3

ASTRONOMICAL COMPASS

Diagram taken from a reproduction of the work entitled *The Golden Mirror of the Art of Healing* (18th century A.D.).

On this astronomical compass the times of day, seasons and their interrelationships are shown as follows:

1. "The Natural Order of Things" (innermost circle).

2. The twelve terrestrial cyclic signs and the division into hours.

3. The relationships of the five elements to each other, and their qualities.

4. The connection between the ten celestial cyclic signs and the elements.

5. The favorable and unfavorable constellations.

33

Healing attempts to explain away the *Yin-Yang* principle and the doctrine of the five elements as a synthesis of philosophy and actual practice. The traditional theses reveal a "simple, materialistic view of antiquity," although this view was not able to embrace all natural phenomena completely into one system— which in any case cannot in all fairness be asked of it.[22]

Kuo Mo-jo writes as follows in his *Book of Tenfold Criticism:* "By virtue of its very origin, such concepts—namely, *Yin-Yang* and the five elements—are opposed to superstition or, to put it more precisely, are scientific." It is as yet too early, however, to make any over-hasty generalizations, as these concepts must be more closely analyzed and more fully substantiated.[23]

The Soviet Professor W. G. Wogralik also demands that more value should be placed on the good, usable theses, whereas a critical attitude should be adopted towards the more antiquated doctrines. Only by this means will it be possible to come to terms with the findings of modern science.[24] The *Yin-Yang* principle and the five elements played an important part in the traditional art of healing, but, because these concepts were handed down in historical documents, their interpretation is difficult and they cannot easily be incorporated into modern medical science. Professor Wogralik therefore believes it necessary for such historical theses to be reworded into scientific language in order to make them more understandable.[25]

MAN AND CLIMATE

The traditional art of healing stresses the importance of investigating climatic influences and their connection with various illnesses. Ever since ancient times an interrelationship has been observed between climate, seasons, and variations in temperature on the one hand, and a balanced state of bodily health on the other. "In spring and summer the *Yin* is weak and the *Yang* dominates; in winter the *Yin* is stronger than the *Yang*," says the 'Ling Shu."[26] According to the "Su Wên," spring is the season of increasing vitality, fecundity in Nature, the time of restitution. During this period the liver can suffer harm if Man does not

34

adjust himself to the natural order of things. Summer is the time when celestial and terrestrial forces combine. Particularly characteristic of this season are cardiac diseases and "the intermittent fever" (malaria). In autumn the forces between heaven and earth balance out, and this season can be harmful for the lungs. Finally, winter is the period when Nature rests and it is now that kidney diseases frequently occur.[27] It was also noted that windy weather in spring caused diarrhea and that summer heat brought on feverish illnesses. The autumnal dampness coincided with "coughing" and the winter cold with feverish ailments which broke out in spring.[28]

These examples show how strangely such observations, accumulated over thousands of years, are mingled with theory. A similar example is to be found in the "Su-Wên," in the section dealing with the effects of taste: ". . . if someone eats many salty things, then his veins become 'stiff and delicate' and the color of his skin changes. If he eats many bitter things, then his skin dries up and he loses his hair. If he eats many pungent things, then he will suffer muscular pains and his nails will atrophy. And, finally, if he eats many sweet things, his 'bones' will be painful and his hair will fall out. These are the injuries caused by the five qualities of taste."[29]

In order to establish how much truth there is in such theories it is essential to have some knowledge of the prevailing climate conditions. China comprises a vast area, and the climate is different from that of Europe. Even the northern, southern, eastern, and western parts of the country differ from one another in respect of climate. It is thus very difficult in many cases to evaluate the knowledge which has been handed down and to discover the empirical core of the matter.

The various ways in which the air moves also have differing effects on the human organism. The "Ling Shu" mentions the spring east wind, the summer south wind, the autumn west wind, and the winter north wind.[30] Thus it was established that the north wind is, generally speaking, a swirling one, with a cleansing effect. The south wind generally blows horizontally and thus carries impurities away with it. It was also observed that the refreshing effect of the cold wind is due to intense stimulation of the skin. It has further been established that colds are caused by one side of the body being cooled down by small imperceptible currents of air. Damp, draughty cold can encourage rheumatic ailments.[31]

The traditional Chinese art of healing attributes the exogenous causes of an illness to wind, cold, draught, dampness, fire, and heat. The wind can cause headache, colds, "stuffed-up noses," and coughs. Cold brings arthralgia, vomiting, diarrhea, and colic. Draught, on the other hand, causes sore throats, coughing, profuse perspiration, and thoracic complaints. Dampness produces tumors, malaria, jaundice, and arthralgia. "Fire" brings sunstroke, heat-strokes, and the spitting of blood. Heat can also cause diarrhea, vomiting, and headache. "Fire" can be taken as meaning a feverish condition. Wind, cold, draught, dampness, and heat can also cause "fire," that is to say, fever. According to the traditional concepts, the "bad winds" chiefly coincide with spring, cold with winter, heat with summer, dampness with "late summer," but draught with autumn.[32]

Modern medicine is also investigating the effect of atmospheric and meteorological conditions on the human organism. It has been proved that the number of breaths people draw varies with the time of year; in Europe the maximum number occurs in January/February and the minimum in July/August. The quantity of hemoglobin is highest in July and least in January. Scientists link these phenomena with the varying intensity of the sun's radiation. This would also appear to be strengthened by the established fact that the number of red blood corpuscles decreases in the case of people who spend long periods in the dark. The thyroid gland contains less iodine and thyroxin (the thyroid gland hormone) in winter than in summer.[33]

There are also significant links between illnesses and the seasons. The organism is particularly vulnerable in spring. The irritability of the autonomic nervous system increases; the phosphorus content of the blood rises, while its calcium content falls. That is why tetany sufferers tend to have convulsive attacks during the first sunny days in spring. (Tetany is a disease associated with increased susceptibility to cramp on the part of the organism; its immediate cause can be traced to a reduction in the calcium content of the blood.) In winter the ultraviolet radiation is reduced and, as a result, the vitamin D content of

36

the organism. Vitamin D controls the calcareous deposits in the bones. It has been established that embolic diseases increase at the end of the winter. Some investigators attribute this to the fact that the iodine content of the blood decreases during winter but suddenly rises in spring, thus abruptly worsening the condition of any patient suffering from hyperfunction of the thyroid gland.[34]

Some groups of illnesses tend to occur more frequently at certain times of year; for example, some forms of pneumonia, meningitis, inflammation of the mucous membrane in the respiratory passages, varicella, whooping-cough, and certain forms of eczema are typical of the winter and spring months; the illnesses typical of the summer and autumn months are intestinal catarrh among infants, typhus, dysentery, and poliomyelitis.[35]

The sequence of weather fronts, too, that is, changes of temperature, air pressure, humidity, and radiation, affect the state of health of people who are susceptible to weather conditions. Science has established that, in the case of people who are sensitive to the arrival of cold fronts, neuralgia, mental instability, high blood pressure, apoplexy, and rheumatic pains occur more frequently. It is also a well-known fact that the number of influenza cases increases when there is a sudden rise in temperature. A cold wind can cause cramp, whereas a warm one has a relaxing effect.

If we compare these modern observations with the findings which the Chinese art of healing has etablished over thousands of years, we can see that, as far as climatic conditions in the Far East are concerned, they approximate basically to actual fact.

3

THE HUMAN BODY
IN ANCIENT CHINESE THOUGHT

So far we have surveyed those works which are regarded in China as forming the mainstay of the old art of healing. We have also dealt with those theses which seek to explain the harmony between Man and Nature.

There were two predominant schools of thought in the traditional art of healing. The one placed the main emphasis on philosophical analysis of the basic concepts and in so doing became further and further divorced from actual practice. We can see this trend in the field of "monastic" medicine, where we find chiefly those Taoist physicians and alchemists who by means of pedantic, literal interpretation sought a solution to the secrets of Nature, attempted to "conquer Nature," and tried to find the source of eternal life. There are numerous references both in Chinese history books and in *belles-lettres* to the successes of such alchemists. In the historical work entitled *Wei Chih,* for example, we read of a Taoist magician who called on the sick to go down on their knees before him and confess their sins. He would then give them water to drink in which a "magic charm" had been dissolved. The essential factor was that the patient should believe in the *Tao.* If he recovered, it was basically due to his belief; if he died, then he had to ascribe it to his own lack of faith.[36]

The other school of medical thought was the art of healing founded on empiricism. Although it is difficult to draw an exact line of differentiation between this doctrine and the monastic art of healing, we may regard it nevertheless as being of common, popular origin. This "folk" knowledge dates back for several thousands of years and it is still very much alive in modern China. Probably every family knew, and still knows, special methods of curing various complaints. The People's Republic of China considers the collection of such "family traditions" to be highly important, and the results of research show that many excellent medicaments and cures have been preserved and handed down from father to son. Many families have now divulged to medical science their scrupulously guarded secrets concerning, for example, medicinal herbs and medicaments for use against snake bites; these remedies are now being tested by modern and traditional doctors working in collaboration and have often met with outstanding success.

Due also to the rich inheritance of acupuncture, medical laymen today know the specific peculiarities of various points on the body which are not even mentioned in much anatomical literature. Such knowledge is, of course, mostly purely empirical, and the surviving commentaries are often fragmentary and tendentious. The Chinese, perhaps as early as the Stone Age, discovered points on the human body which, if pressed or punctured, helped to alleviate pain or produced other effects. (The Chinese Stone Age is considerably later than the European one, however. In North China the Bronze Age did not begin till the second millennium B.C.; in South China the Stone Age persisted through the 3rd and 2nd centuries B.C.).

The existence of stone needles helps to support the theory that acupuncture evolved during the Stone Age. Stone needles were, of course, also used for surgical operations. It was also known, even in the earliest times, that burning or heating certain points on the body increases full-bloodedness and alleviates pain. These processes were later used to more purposeful effect.[37]

The pressing and rubbing of painful and diseased parts of the body, together with attempts to revive newly born infants, may be regarded as the predecession of systematic massage.

The changing rhythm of breathing and the accompanying tightening and loosening of the muscles as well as subsequent changes in the organism, became evident during the ecstasy of the shaman dances. This perhaps formed the basis for the subsequent systematization of respiratory exercises.

It is difficult to decide which of the various methods of healing came first in order of time. It is thought probable that the use of stone implements and, therefore, of stone needles preceded that of fire, so that acupuncture by means of stone needles would be older than healing by moxibustion.[38] It is also known that the present form of physiotherapy is of later origin. The various traditional healing processes originated in different parts of China, so that we may assume that the individual experiences originally depended on regional conditions.

Let us return to the use of stone needles. In antique China, in times which can no longer be historically defined, it had been discovered that there are certain points on the body which, if punctured or burned, had a beneficial effect on certain ailments. Through the exchange and widening of experience more and more points were discovered, by means of which it was possible not only to alleviate pain but also to influence the functioning of certain internal organs.[39] Traditional medical literature reveals that the number of such points on the body kept increasing with the passage of time. They were arranged in order of degree, first, second and third, and new connections kept being discovered between the various points and the internal organs.[40] In order to make them more easily remembered the points were given names. In accordance with the spirit of the times this nomenclature was only partly anatomical.

These so-called acupuncture points are symmetrically distributed over both halves of the body. The "Su Wên" and the "Ling Shu" list a total of 295 (according to other sources, 365) points. Huang-fu Mi refers to 649 points. The bronze figure of the Sung period lists 657. The medical work entitled *Compendium of Acupuncture and Moxibustion* (*Chên-chiu Ta-ch'êng*), compiled during the Ming period, describes 667 points. Today some 722 points are generally acknowledged.[41]

Of particular importance is the fact that numerous widely separated points affect the functioning of one and the same organ. This finding was already noted in *The Yellow Emperor's Classic of Internal Medicine*. All points which affect the same

40

organ were later found to be interconnected, and these inter-connections were given the name *Ching,* that is to say, me-ridians.[42] The original number of meridians was twelve, but two more were added later. There were, however, other points apart from these connecting lines which could not be thus classified, and these were subsequently entitled the *eight special meridians.* The first two of these are the two which we already mentioned, namely, the additions to the original twelve. Other points, func-tioning in a similar manner, were combined to form the *twelve extra meridians.* In addition, a list was made of those points which affect, not the internal organs, but the skin and the muscles, and these were called the *muscular meridians.*

All of these meridians have a definite functional character, de-pending on whether they affect organs, muscles, or skin. Knowl-edge of the interconnection between the surface of the skin and the internal organs is the unique and special discovery of ancient Chinese medicine.

These points and meridians are found both on human bodies and on those of animals. This knowledge also dates back thousands of years and features largely in books on veterinary surgery. Today, as in days gone by, veterinary surgeons use heated needles and moxibustion. This testifies to recognition of the fundamental fact that there is no basic difference between the organism of human beings and that of animals, particularly vertebrates.[43]

We have already noted the fact that traditional Chinese medi-cine divides the internal organs into two large groups, the "storage" (passive) and "working" (active). In terms of the *Yin-Yang* principle the "storage" organs are called *Yin* organs and the "working" ones *Yang* organs. In Chinese the *Yin* organs are called *"Tsang,"* and the *Yang* organs are called *"Fu."* Thus we get the following classification of organs:

Passive, "storage" Yin organs (Tsang's)	Active, "working" Yang organs (Fu's)
lungs	large intestine
spleen	stomach
heart	small intestine
kidneys	urinary bladder
liver	gall bladder

41

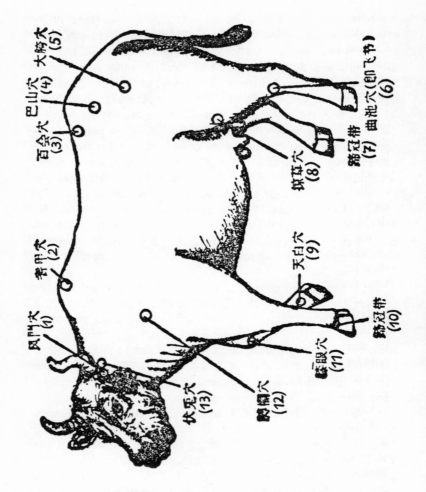

風門穴 (1)
督門穴 (2)
百会穴 (3)
巴山穴 (4)
大胯穴 (5)
曲池穴(即飞节) (6)
蹄冠带 (7)
蹲亚穴 (8)
天臼穴 (9)
蹄冠带 (10)
姜眼穴 (11)
网�`穴 (12)
伏兔穴 (13)

FIGURE 4
ACUPUNCTURE POINTS
IN VETERINARY SCIENCE
The most important points on the body of a cow. The drawing is taken from a Chinese veterinary science periodical. The circles denote the individual points while the characters are their names: 1. *Fêng-mên* point; 2. *Ch'i-chia* point; 3. *Pai-hui* point; 4. *Pa-shan* point; 5. *Ta-k'ua* point; 6. *Chü-ch'ih* point; 7. point in the upper area of the hoof; 8. *Liao-ts'ao* point; 9. *T'ien-pai* point; 10. point in the upper area of the hoof; 11. *Hsi-yen* point; 12. *Po-lan* point; 13. *Fu-t'u* point.

42

Later the "organ" called the "controller of the heart" was included in the *Tsang* group. (The literal translation from the Chinese of "controller of the heart" is "heart sinus," though this has nothing in common with the modern anatomical term "heart sinus" or pericardium.) The "controller of the heart" denotes a functional cycle of the peripheral part of the blood circulation.

Among the *Fu* organs is the one referred to as the "triple warmer," by which is meant the functional cycle which controls the chemical environment of the organism, comprised of the interaction of respiration, digestion, and the urogenital system. It represents the body's main source of energy.

On the other hand, the "controller of the heart" regulates not only the peripheral blood circulation but also the composition of the blood and the supply of blood to the *Yin* organs.[44]

The traditional medical view was that the individual organs are closely linked as regards function. The modern idea is that they form part of the structure of the autonomic nervous system. As far as bodily energy is concerned, they are like the links in a chain; thus the liver is linked to the lungs, the lungs to the large intestine, the large intestine to the stomach, the stomach to the spleen, the spleen to the heart, the heart to the small intestine, the small intestine to the urinary bladder, the urinary bladder to the kidneys, the kidneys to the circulation, the circulation to the "triple warmer," the latter to the gall bladder, and the gall bladder to the liver, thus completing the cycle. (See the following diagram.)

Under this arrangement the *Yin* and *Yang* organs belong together in pairs: liver and lungs are *Yin,* large intestine and stomach *Yang,* spleen and heart *Yin,* small intestine and urinary bladder *Yang,* kidneys and circulation *Yin,* the "triple warmer" and the gall-bladder *Yang.*[45] Let us now see how far this idea corresponds with actual fact.

liver	lungs
gall bladder	large intestine
"triple warmer"	stomach
"controller of the heart"	spleen
kidneys	heart
urinary bladder	small intestine

Traditional medical science has found that, as far as tonification and sedation of the organic functions are concerned, the most effective treatments are those which not only affect the meridian and the points belonging to the particular organ, but which also (in the case of tonification) stimulate the preceding organ and (in the case of sedation) affect the organ which follows it in the sequence. To make this point clearer we must first of all explain the relationship between organs and meridians.

The old medical experts discovered that there were functional links between certain meridians and organs. The names of the meridians are derived from this fact. The meridians affecting the hands and feet run either in a centrifugal direction, that is, from the organ in question to the limbs, or in a centripetal direction, from the limbs to the relevant organs. The meridians which run on the inside of the arms and the legs are called *Yin* meridians, those on the outside the *Yang* meridians. Thus on the inside of each arm and leg there are three meridians belonging to the six *Yin* organs, and similarly there are three meridians on the outside of each arm and leg corresponding to the six *Yang* organs. In order, perhaps, to enable these groups of three to be more easily remembered they were further subdivided into *Yin* and *Yang* meridians with strong, medium, and weak "energy." It is not possible to say as yet whether or not this subdivision corresponds with actual fact.

For one thing, Chinese and Western interpretations are at variance here. Of the well-known Western acupuncture research experts, Soulié de Morant describes this division as a mere matter of nomenclature,[46] while Chamfrault must have presumably construed the names wrongly, since he translates the term *Shao-Yang* (= little *Yang*) by *"iang moyen"* (= medium *Yang*), and the term *Yang-Ming* (= light of *Yang*) by *"iang inférieur"* (= weak *Yang*).[47] Another leading Western author, G. Bachmann, adopts Chamfrault's translation of *Shao-Yang* (= little *Yang*) as *"medium Yang."*[48] For the sake of clarity we shall therefore dispense with the nomenclature of *Yin* and *Yang* according to their degrees of energy.

The meridians can be classified as follows:

Yin meridians on the inside of the arms	lung meridian "controller of the heart" meridian heart meridian

Yang meridians on the outside of the arms	small intestine meridian
	"triple warmer" meridian
	large intestine meridian
Yin meridians on the inside of the legs	spleen meridian
	kidney meridian
	liver meridian
Yang meridians on the oustide of the legs	urinary bladder meridian
	gall bladder meridian
	stomach meridian

Under this arrangement the meridian of an organ is composed of all the points on the body by which the organ in question is primarily affected. We must, however, consider the individual organs within the context as a whole. For example, the points of the stomach meridian include some which affect the mouth, gullet, stomach lining, and so on. The lung meridian consists of points affecting the nose, windpipe, bronchia, lung vesicles, and others.

Not all points of a meridian are equally effective. Both the traditional Chinese works and the European literature on the subject grade them according to their degree of importance. We shall return to this subject later.

TONIFICATION AND SEDATION, AND THE IMPORTANT ACUPUNCTURE POINTS

The *Tsang* and *Fu* vessels which we have already mentioned are interconnected; through them passes what traditional medical science calls "energy" (*Ch'i*). *Ch'i* originally meant "air" or "breath," so that it derives from a very ancient concept. In his *Reflections* (*Lun Hêng*) of the materialistic philosopher Wang Ch'ung, who lived from 27 to 95 A.D., *Ch'i* already signified the original material substance, the "original nebula" or prime energy which motivates the *Tao,* or law of nature, as the principle of development behind all phenomena. This "energy" circulates through the entire body; it regulates the circulation of the blood, ingestion, and the autoprotection of the organism. It also flows along the meridians. If it is hindered from circulating or blocked as the result of some external or endogenous circumstance, an abnormal surplus or lack of energy results, and not only in the organ which is linked to the meridian in question; the whole harmony of the entire organism is upset—and a condition of illness is present.

If the functioning of an organ begins to fail, it must be strengthened; on the other hand, in the event of hyperfunction the excess of "energy" must, as it were, be drawn off. Thus tonification and sedation imply that harmony can be restored through the application of stimulating or subduing treatment at the relevant points on the body. In other words, tonification represents "strong, persistent stimulation," whereas sedation means a weak, calming influence.

In Chinese medical works the acupuncture points on the body are divided into the following main groups.[49]

1. The *Mu* points: these are situated in the vicinity of the diseased parts but lie on a meridian which does not belong to the same organ. (Bachmann calls these "alarm points."[50])

2. The *Ching* points: these are at the beginning and end of the meridians.

3. The points of tonification and sedation.

4. The *Lo* points, which equalize the "energy" between the meridians that are interconnected according to the *Yin-Yang* principle, for example between the lung and large intestine meridians. (Bachmann calls these "passage points."[51])

5. The *Yü* points (also referred to as "approval or associated points") are located on the bladder meridian which runs along both sides of the spinal column. According to Bachmann, they should be regarded as being segment-dependent, and they may well be connected with the innervation of the spinal cord segments.[52]

6. The points, found on all meridians, which correspond to the five elements: the *Ching* points (wood element), the *Yung* points (fire element), the *Yüan* and *Yü* points (earth element), the *Ching* points—in Chinese written with different characters from the one above—(metal element), and the *Ho* points (water element). All these are located along the meridians which are linked with the *Yin* organs.

The following points are found on the *Yang* organs and their associated meridians: the *Ching* points (metal element), the

46

Yung points (water element), the *Yü* and *Yüan* points (wood element), the *Ching* points (fire element), and the *Ho* points (earth element).[53]

7. The "special points" are normally brought into play in the case of special illnesses, for example circulatory disorders or for tonification or sedation of the vagus nerve, and so on.

Now let us take a closer look at each of these groups:

1. The *Mu* or "alarm points" are located on the front of the trunk, but not at the extremities. Stimulation of the *Mu* points has an instantaneous effect. Every meridian except that at the circulation has a *Mu* point.

2. The beginnings and end points of each meridian enable a harmonization of the entire organism.

3. The tonification and sedation points are perhaps the most important of all. Here we must refer once again to the empirical division in accordance with the five elements. The traditional art of healing arranged these points in order of effectiveness and grouped the five elements accordingly. According to the rule referred to as the "mother and son," an illness caused by an excessive function, that is to say, one of a hyperfunctional nature, was treated by means of sedation of the affected organ and, at the same time, by applying tranquillizing treatment to the organ next in sequence in the "energy cycle"; thus both the organ itself and its "son" were treated. For example, in the event of a hyperfunctional disorder of the "pulmonary tract," the "son," as well as the points of the lung meridian, have to be given sedation. Since the lungs belong to the *Yin* group of the metal element, and this is followed by the water element, the *Ho* point, which is linked to the water element, must be tranquillized as well.

If, on the other hand, a disorder of the pulmonary tract occurs as the result of hypofunction, then not only must the functioning of the pulmonary tract, which belongs to the metal element, be stimulated, but also the "mother." In preceding order this is the *Yü* point of the earth element. The naming of the points according to the elements is only of secondary importance and actually serves merely to make practical implementation more easy to grasp.[54]

4. The *Lo* or "passage points" are likely meant for the

achievement of harmony. Subdivision according to the five elements means that each element has a *Yin* and a *Yang* organ. For example:

fire element:	*Yin* = heart	*Yang* = small intestine
earth element:	*Yin* = spleen	*Yang* = stomach
metal element:	*Yin* = lungs	*Yang* = large intestine
water element:	*Yin* = kidneys	*Yang* = bladder
wood element:	*Yin* = liver	*Yang* = gall bladder

This division also includes the functional cycles of the "controller of the heart" and the "triple warmer." Both belong to the fire element. The "controller" is *Yin,* whereas the "triple warmer" is *Yang.* It was observed that *Yin-Yang* pairs belonging to the same element were often interrelated. If the one organ was in a condition of hyperfunction, it could mean a functional weakness on the part of the corresponding organ. In order for harmony to be achieved it would be necessary to stimulate the *Lo* point which exercises an equalizing function between the two organs. If, for example, the activity of the gall bladder is too weak, but the functioning of the liver is over-strong, then the *Lo* point of the liver has to be stimulated in order to equalize the organism. If the opposite were the case, then the *Lo* point of the gall bladder meridian would have to be treated.

5. The *Yü* points belong to the sedative category and they exert by nature an equalizing and harmonizing influence. Each organ possesses one of these points. They are located on the bladder meridian on both sides of the spinal column, between the first dorsal vertebra and the last lumbar vertebra. There are twelve *Yü* points, just as there are twelve main meridians.

6 Of the points which correspond to the five elements, the *Yüan* or "source points" are worth mentioning. These are located near the points of tonification and sedation and strengthen their effect.[55] Similar effects can also be achieved by means of the so-called *Ho* or "reunion points." These *Ho* points link the twelve main meridians with other meridians.[56]

7. The "special points" are particularly important in the case of functional disorders. These points are not linked to individual organs, but affect the interplay or *synergy* of all organs. They thus react on the adrenal glands, the connective tissues, haema-

48

poiesis, the balance of the sympathetic nervous system, blood pressure, and so on.

TECHNIQUES FOR TONIFICATION AND SEDATION

1. In the case of hypofunction (*Yin* condition), the following points must be stimulated:
   (a) the stimulation point of the meridian belonging to the organ;
   (b) the *Yüan* or "source point" of the organ;
   (c) the starting point of the meridian belonging to the organ.

2. In the case of hyperfunction (*Yang* condition), sedation can be achieved via the following points:
   (a) the sedation point of the meridian belonging to the organ;
   (b) the *Yüan* or "source point" of the organ;
   (c) the starting point of the meridian belonging to the organ.[57]

The "mother and son" rule already referred to obtains for both spheres of application.

THE MAIN MERIDIANS

In this chapter we propose to describe the meridians, which have already been referred to, together with their location and their relationship to the "cycle of energy." The individual meridians are illustrated by means of diagrams.

The *lung meridian* is a *T'ai-Yin* (= strong *Yin*) meridian running along the arms. According to traditional theory, it obtains its energy from the liver meridian, which is *Yin* in character and is associated with the wood element. It transmits energy to the large intestine meridian, which is *Yang* in character and belongs to the metal element. The lung meridian itself is also allotted to the metal element, and it runs in a "centrifugal" direction. Its starting point is near the armpit between the second and third ribs. It runs along the inside of the upper and lower arm and ends on the inside of the thumb. It links 11 points of the body (22 in all, counting both sides).

It is possible to measure changes in the electropotential values along this meridian in cases of abnormal disorders of the respiratory system, such as bronchial catarrh, inflammation of the lungs, asthmatic complaints, and angina, and also as a result of secondary phenomena due to heart diseases and certain nose and eye ailments.[58]

The *heart meridian* is likewise *Yin* in character (*Shao-Yin* = little *Yin*) and is associated with the fire element. According to traditional theory, it obtains its energy from the spleen meridian, which is likewise *Yin* in character but belongs to the earth element; and transmits energy to the small intestine meridian, which is *Yang* in character and is associated with the fire element. The heart meridian runs in a "centrifugal" direction; its starting point is located beneath the chest muscle (*musculus pectoralis*) at the level of the third rib. It runs along the inside of the upper and lower arms and ends on the inside of the top section of the little finger, near the corner of the nail fold.

This meridian links 9 points of the body (18 in all, counting both sides). Fluctuating electropotential values indicate heart disease and circulatory disorders. Secondary phenomena, such as diseases of the small intestine, larynx, and eyes, are also

---

FIGURE 5

THE LUNG MERIDIAN AND ITS SPHERE OF INFLUENCE

The dotted black line denotes the link to the internal organs and the continuous black line the meridian itself. The figures and arrows show the course of the meridian. (The 12 main meridians shown in the following diagrams, together with the special meridians *Tu-mai* and *Jên-mai*, are depicted in the same way. The illustrations are taken from the Chinese work entitled *A Summary of the Traditional Chinese Art of Healing*.)

Explanation of symbols:

●   acupuncture points of the meridian in question

▲   acupuncture points of other meridians

‒ ‒ ‒   section of the meridian in question leading to organs, without points

——   section of the meridian in question running through the subcutaneous cellular tissue, showing points

·~·~·   internal organs

50

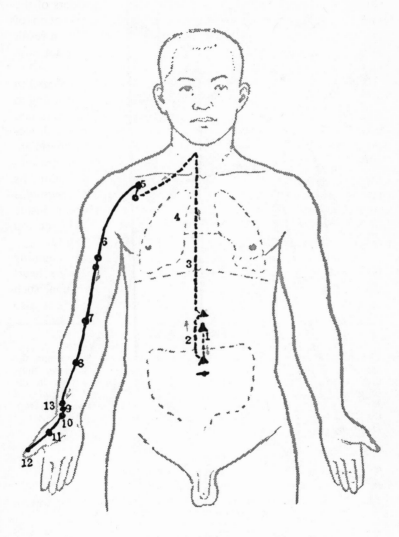

FIGURE 5
THE LUNG MERIDIAN AND ITS SPHERE OF INFLUENCE

51

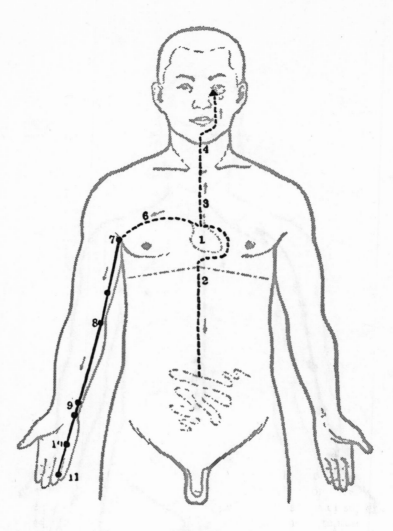

FIGURE 6
THE HEART MERIDIAN AND ITS SPHERE OF INFLUENCE
(For an explanation of symbols see Figure 5.)

registered. The measured values on this meridian are often irregular during the change of life (*climacteric*).[59]

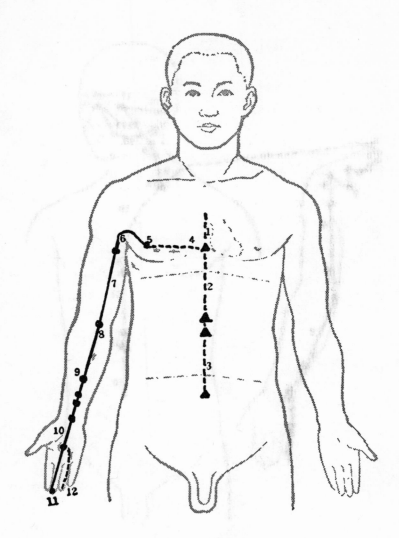

FIGURE 7
THE "CONTROLLER OF THE HEART" MERIDIAN
AND ITS SPHERE OF INFLUENCE
(For an explanation of symbols see Figure 5.)

The "*controller of the heart*" *meridian* is the third which is
Yin in character and traverses the arms (*Chüeh-Yin* = end of

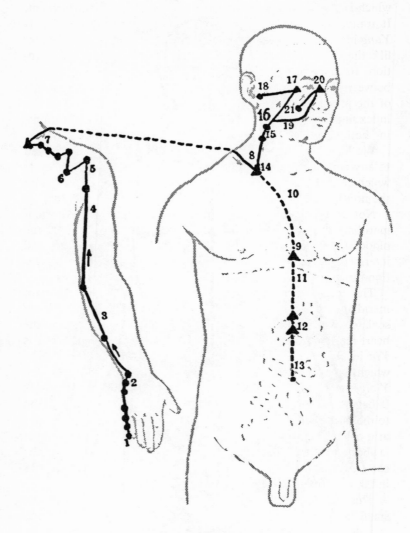

FIGURE 8
THE SMALL INTESTINE MERIDIAN AND ITS SPHERE OF INFLUENCE
(For an explanation of symbols see Figure 5.)

Yin); it is associated with the fire element. According to traditional theory, it obtains its energy from the kidney meridian,

which is also *Yin* in character but belongs to the water element. It transmits energy to the "triple warmer" meridian, which is *Yang* in character and belongs to the fire element. This meridian, like the two just mentioned, also runs in a "centrifugal" direction. Its starting point lies between the nipple and the armpit, between the third and fourth ribs. It, too, runs along the inside of the arm and ends on the inside of the upper section of the index finger. It comprises 9 acupuncture points (18 in all, counting both sides).

We have already mentioned that this meridian is not linked to any particular organ, but that it represents a functional cycle which determines the peripheral circulation, the blood count, and the nourishment of the *Yin* organs.

Not enough research has been carried out on this important meridian as yet. According to Bachmann, it is linked to the blood stream and all its endocrine, serological components and intermediary metabolic products. This also includes the oxydation processes.[60]

The *small intestine meridian* belongs to the *Yang* group of meridians on the arms (*T'ai-Yang* = strong *Yang*) and is associated with the fire element. It receives its energy from the heart meridian, which likewise belongs to the fire element but is *Yin* in character. It transmits energy to the bladder meridian, which is connected with the water element and belongs to the *Yang* meridians. It runs in a "centripetal" direction to the trunk. It begins above the end of the nail of the little finger, runs on to the dorsal side of the forearm, along the *ulna,* over the upper arm to the shoulder joint, and thence across the neck and lower jawbone to the outer corner of the eye. It ends in front of the ear (*lobulus auriculae*). It connects 19 points of the body (38 in all, counting both sides).

This meridian reflects the healthy or disturbed state of the small intestine. Functional disorders of the stomach and heart can also be measured by means of it. Irregularities in the "energy cycle" of the meridian also occur in cases of neurasthenia, psychosis, Parkinsonism, and epilepsy.[61]

The *"triple warmer" meridian* is *Yang* in character (*Shao-Yang* = little *Yang*) and belongs to the fire element. It receives its *energy* from the *circulation meridian,* which likewise belongs to the fire element but is *Yin* in character. It transmits energy to the gall bladder meridian, which belongs to the wood element and is *Yang* in character. It runs in a "centripetal" direction. Its starting point lies above the nail of the ring finger. It runs up the dorsal side of the arm across the shoulder to the clavicle, rises from here to the bone of the temple, circles the ear, goes down to the lower jawbone, and ends at the outer corner of the eye. It comprises 23 points of the body (46 in all, counting both sides).

As we have already stated, this meridian is not linked to any definite organs. According to traditional theory, it consists of three sections, the lower, central, and upper "warmers." The upper one controls respiration, the central one regulates the complex functions of digestion and ingestion, while the lower one affects the urogenital system, sexual potency, and the chemical state of the whole organism. The "triple warmer" represents a controlling functional cycle which, by virtue of its opposing actions, counterbalances the function of the "controller of the heart." Any disturbances of its functioning may be accompanied by disorders of the respiratory passages, together with convulsions, deafness, and neuralgia.[62]

The *large intestine meridian* is *Yang* in character (*Yang-Ming* = light of the *Yang*) and belongs to the metal element. It receives its energy from the lung meridian, which belongs to the metal element also but is *Yin* in character. It transmits energy to the stomach meridian, which is *Yang* in character and belongs to the earth element. This meridian, like the previous two, runs in a "centripetal" direction. Its starting point is on the outer side of the top section of the index finger, near the nail root. From there it runs along the outer ventral side of the arm to the clavicle. It touches the upper cervical vertebrae, turns there, and goes back to the clavicle, though more in the vicinity of the breastbone. It then runs via the lower jawbone and the corner of the mouth to the opposite nasolabial fold, where it ends. This meridian links 20 points on the body (40 in all, counting both sides). Appreciable changes in this meridian mainly reflect diseases of the large intestine, but also secondary ailments af-

56

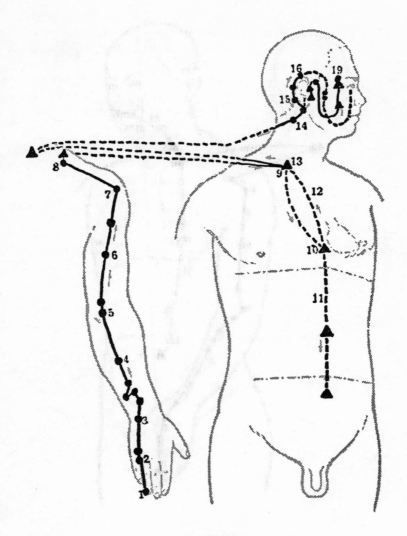

FIGURE 9

THE "TRIPLE WARMER" MERIDIAN AND ITS SPHERE OF INFLUENCE
(For an explanation of symbols see Figure 5.)

fecting the teeth and gums, asthmatic complaints, and various skin diseases.[63]

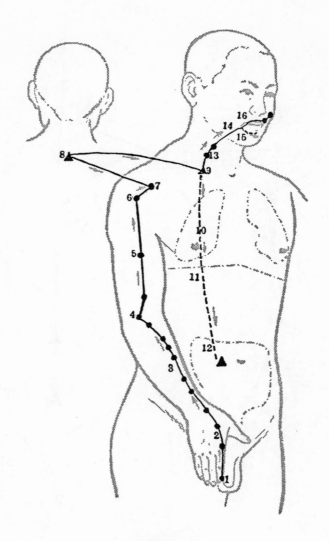

FIGURE 10
THE LARGE INTESTINE MERIDIAN AND ITS SPHERE OF INFLUENCE
(For an explanation of symbols see Figure 5.)

The *spleen meridian* is *Yin* in character and is associated with
the earth element. It obtains its energy from the stomach

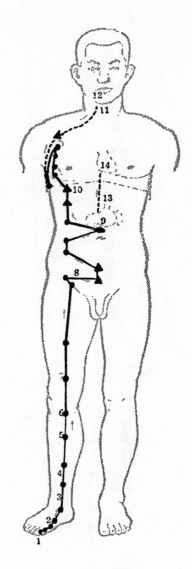

FIGURE II
THE SPLEEN MERIDIAN AND ITS SPHERE OF INFLUENCE
(For an explanation of symbols see Figure 5.)

59

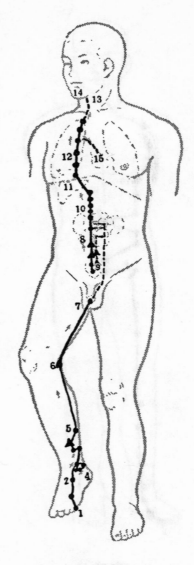

FIGURE 12
THE KIDNEY MERIDIAN AND ITS SPHERE OF INFLUENCE
(For an explanation of symbols see Figure 5.)

60

meridian, which belongs to the earth element but is *Yang* in character, and transmits it to the *heart meridian* which is associated with the fire element and is *Yin* in character. The starting point of this meridian is on the outside of the upper section of the big toe, whence it runs along the inside of the leg, touching the area of the navel, thence obliquely past the nipple until it ends in the vicinity of the second intercostal space. It runs in a "centripetal" direction and includes 21 points (42 in all, counting both sides).[64]

Bachmann calls this the spleen-pancreas meridian, and not the spleen meridian.[65] Chinese sources and Western publications are at variance here regarding the assumed course of this meridian (see the books which we have quoted by Bachmann and Chamfrault).

Appreciable changes in this meridian are associated with irregularities in digestion and sugar content of the body, temperamental changes, and allergic and convulsive conditions.

The *kidney meridian* is *Yin* in character (*Shao-Yin* = little *Yin*) and is associated with the water element. It receives its energy from the bladder meridian, which likewise belongs to the water element but is *Yang* in character; and transmits energy to the circulation meridian, which is *Yin* in character and belongs to the fire element. This meridian runs in a "centripetal" direction. It begins on the sole of the front part of the foot, runs along the inside of the lower leg and the thigh up to the area of the bladder, thence past the navel and breastbone and ends on the ends on the sternal side of the clavicle. It comprises 27 points (54 in all, counting both sides).

Appreciable changes in this meridian can be due to kidney and heart irregularities of circulation and to conditions of a neurasthenic and epileptic nature.[66]

The *liver meridian* is the third of those which begin in the area of the legs. It is *Yin* in character (*Chüeh-Yin* = end of *Yin*) and associated with the wood element. According to traditional teaching, it receives its energy from the gall bladder meridian, which likewise belongs to the wood element but is *Yang* in character. It transmits its energy to the lung meridian, which is *Yin* in character and belongs to the metal element.

This "centripetal" meridian starts between the big and second

61

toes, runs along the inside of the lower leg and thigh, past the groin and bladder, touches the floating ribs, and ends near the nipple. It consists of 14 points of the body (28 in all, counting both sides).

Appreciable changes in this meridian can reflect jaundice, vegetative symptoms of fatigue, swelling of the liver, and intestinal disorders, together with secondary effects such as emaciation, allergies, headaches, and arthralgia.[67]

The *bladder meridian* also begins in the area of the legs, but is *Yang* in character (*T'ai-Yang* = strong *Yang*) and is associated with the water element. According to traditional theory, it receives its energy from the small intestine meridian, which is *Yang* in character and associated with the fire element. It transmits energy to the kidney meridian, which is *Yin* in character and belongs to the water element.

Its starting point is at the inner corner of the eye, whence it runs across the vault of the cranium; at the neck it divides into two strands which run down the back in parallel, touching the area of the coccyx. One strand reaches the heel by way of the dorsal center of the leg and ends on the lower section of the little toe. The second ends in the hollow of the knee. This meridian thus runs "centrifugally" and touches 67 points (134 in all, counting both sides).

Appreciable changes in this meridian may denote painful, convulsive conditions, headaches, neuralgia, rheumatic pains, sciatica, and lumbago, and secondary effects such as metabolic disorders of the cells, eczema, and disturbances in the water content of the body.[68]

The *gall bladder meridian* also touches the legs; it is *Yang* in character (*Shao-Yang* = little *Yang*), associated with the wood element, and receives its energy from the "triple warmer" meridian, which is also *Yang* in character but associated with the fire element. It transmits energy to the liver meridian, which is *Yin* in character and associated with the wood element. It runs in a "centrifugal" direction. Beginning at the outer corner of the eye, it runs across the temples and the occipital zone to the central part of the trapezius muscle, thence obliquely past the shoulder joint to the top of the pelvis and along the outside of the leg to the lower section of the fourth toe.

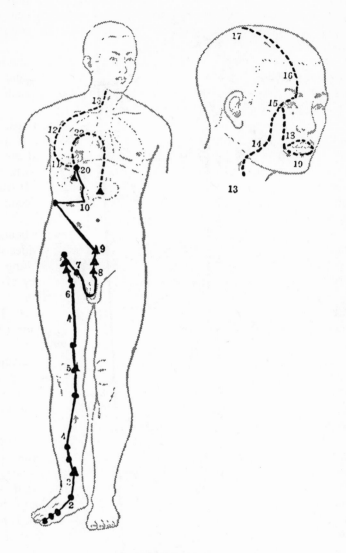

FIGURE 13

THE LIVER MERIDIAN AND ITS SPHERE OF INFLUENCE

The diagram (top, right) depicts the section of the meridian which is in the head. (For an explanation of symbols see Figure 5.)

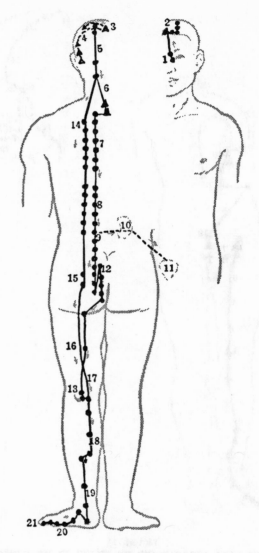

FIGURE 14
THE BLADDER MERIDIAN AND ITS SPHERE OF INFLUENCE
(For an explanation of symbols see Figure 5.)

64

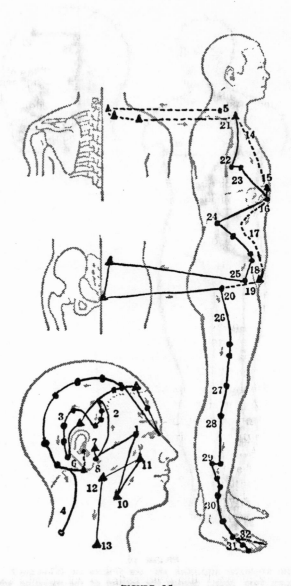

FIGURE 15

THE GALL BLADDER MERIDIAN AND ITS SPHERE OF INFLUENCE

The diagram (*Bottom left*) depicts the section of the meridian which is in the head. (For an explanation of symbols see Figure 5.)

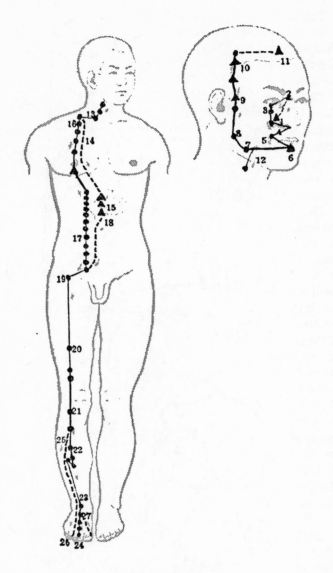

FIGURE 16
THE STOMACH MERIDIAN AND ITS SPHERE OF INFLUENCE
The diagram (top, right) depicts the section of the meridian which is
in the head. (For an explanation of symbols see Figure 5.)

66

This meridian links 44 points (88 in all, counting both sides).

As this meridian is influenced by *Yang,* any appreciable changes therein are associated with pain, such as, for example, migraine, convulsive conditions of the sense organs, and, particularly, pains in the lower limbs and neuralgia.[69]

The *stomach meridian* is the third which touches the legs; it is *Yang* in character (*Yang-Ming* = light of *Yang*) and is connected with the earth element. It receives its energy from the large intestine meridian, which is also *Yang* in character but belongs to the metal element; and transmits energy to the spleen meridian, which is *Yin* in character and associated with the earth element.

The stomach meridian also runs in a "centrifugal" direction. It begins at the nasolabial fold, runs along the lower jawbone to the vicinity of the temples, and thence back to the lower jawbone; it then runs via the clavicle and nipple and past the navel to the vicinity of the hip, whence it goes along the front of the thigh and lower leg till it ends on the top section of the second toe. It connects 45 points (90 in all, counting both sides).

Changes in the area of this meridian are caused by disorders of the stomach and digestive tract, by secondary convulsive conditions of the facial muscles (tics), and by painful conditions of the cervical muscles.[70]

We cannot go into more detail here about the individual points of the body on these twelve meridians or their importance or the illnesses which can be diagnosed by the change in electropotential at these points, since that would go beyond the scope of this book. We shall merely point out that the position of some of these points on the meridians, for example, on the stomach, bladder, large intestine, and spleen meridians, is marked differently in Chinese books than in European works. Our study is based on the traditional Chinese works.

Our description of the twelve meridians, and the table below, which shows the relationships between the meridians and *the cycle of energy,*[71] are meant to depict the relationship of the various meridians to the five elements and to the *Yin-Yang* principle, and thus fully elaborate the traditional Chinese concept of tonification and sedation.

67

Meridian	Course	Character	Meridian	Course	Character
liver (wood element)	legs	*Yin*	*lungs* (metal element)	arms	*Yin*
gall bladder (wood element)	legs	*Yang*	*large intestine* (metal element)	arms	*Yang*
"triple warmer" (fire element)	arms	*Yang*	*stomach* (earth element)	legs	*Yang*
circulation (fire element)	arms	*Yin*	*spleen* (earth element)	legs	*Yin*
kidneys (water element)	legs	*Yin*	*heart* (fire element)	arms	*Yin*
bladder (water element)	legs	*Yang*	*small intestine* (fire element)	arms	*Yang*

THE EIGHT SPECIAL MERIDIANS

As early as the 3rd/2nd centuries B.C. the *Book of Ailments* (*Nan Ching*) mentions the existence and importance of the special meridians;[72] their precise description is linked with the name of Li Shih-chên (1518–1593).

But why are these meridians called "special" meridians? (Bachmann even refers to them as "miraculous meridians."[73])

Each of the twelve meridians described in the preceding chapter comprises in particular stimulating and tranquillizing points of the body. The special meridians do not have these points, however. According to the traditional art of healing, there are eight such special meridians:

1. the *Tu-mai meridian* ("governing vessel")
2. the *Jên-mai meridian* ("vessel of conception," *"vaisseau conception"*)[74]
3. the *Ch'ung-mai meridian* ("vessel of the uninhibitor")
4. the *Tai-mai meridian* ("belt vessel")
5. the *Yin-chiao-mai meridian* ("vessel of the *Yin* exciter")
6. the *Yang-chiao-mai meridian* ("vessel of the *Yang* exciter")

68

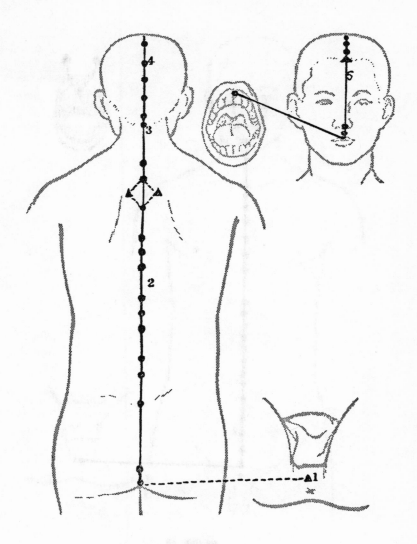

FIGURE 17
THE TU-MAI SPECIAL MERIDIAN
(For an explanation of symbols see Figure 5.)

7. the *Yin-wei-mai meridian* ("vessel of the *Yin* keeper")
8. the *Yang-wei-mai meridian* ("vessel of the *Yang* keeper").

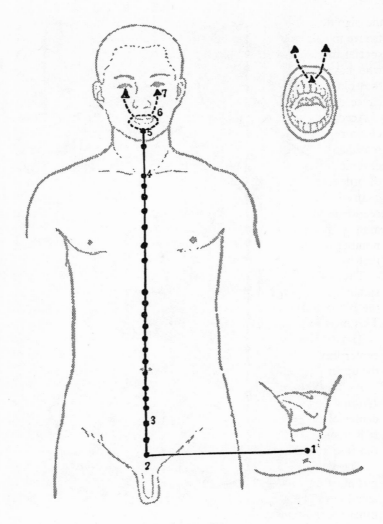

FIGURE 18
THE JÊN-MAI SPECIAL MERIDIAN
(For an explanation of symbols see Figure 5.)

Thus the *Tu-mai, Tai-mai,* and *Yang-chiao-mai* meridians are *Yang* vessels; the *Jên-mai, Ch'ung-mai, Yin-chao-mai,* and *Yin-wei-mai* meridians are *Yin* in character. The old doctors explained

70

the significance of the special meridians by stating that if the twelve main meridians could be regarded as rivers, then the eight special meridians could be compared to lakes or seas. Doctors who have engaged in historical research have also mentioned that old books contain widely differing ideas as to the significance of the special meridians.[75]

According to Bachmann, these eight special "vessels" exercise a regulating function in the event of a blockage in the main meridians. They also play a special part in the treatment of chronic diseases, vegetative conditions of fatigue, metabolic disorders, and psychic strain.[76]

In the course of time, the first two of the eight special meridians, namely the *Tu-mai* and the *Jên-mai,* were counted among the twelve main meridians, thus increasing the latter number to fourteen. We shall now summarize the nature of these first two special meridians.

The *Tu-mai* meridian is *Yang* in character; it runs along the spinal column, one extremity being in the region of the anus, the other being in the mouth, in the gum above the incisors. This meridian links 28 points of the body.[77]

The *Jên-mai meridian* is *Yin* in character; it runs along the center line from chest to abdomen and extends from the gum of the upper jawbone to the region of the anus.

As the *Tu-mai* meridian is *Yang* in character whereas the *Jên-mai* is *Yin;* both of them, running as they do along the center of the body, are associated with the *Yin-Yang* principle. It is assumed that these meridians show appreciable changes in the case of maldevelopment and vegetative dysfunction.

The *Jên-mai* meridian links 24 points, including some important *Mu* points (alarm points) which react on the bladder, small intestine, stomach, and heart and lung meridians. It has no other special points.[78]

Of what value are these special meridians?

The views of Chinese authors are at variance on this point. A book entitled *Summary of the Traditional Chinese Art of Healing (Chung-i-hsiieh Kai-lun[79])* deals only superficially with the eight special meridians and notes that the information which has been handed down represents widely differing views. In other medical works the *Tu-mai* and *Jên-mai* meridians are generally

71

not mentioned till after the twelve main meridians, and the remaining six special meridians are either not mentioned at all or their points are referred to as "special openings outside the meridians."[80]

The publications of Chu Lien and W. G. Wogralik,[81] however, do mention the *Tu-mai* and *Jên-mai* meridians (the *Tu-mai* meridian = 27 points of the body and the *Jên-mai* = 24), but they give no details of their medical significance beyond indicating the precise anatomical locations of these points. Of the European authors, Chamfrault describes the special meridians on the basis of the "Su Wên" and "Ling Shu,"[82] whereas Soulié de Morant does not mention them at all; Bachmann does so as indicated above.

Chu Lien and Wogralik may be correct in merely indicating the position and effect of the points of the body on the special meridians; it seems not out of the question, however, that a scientific investigation into these meridians might lead to a more useful or at least different interpretation.

THE SUBSIDIARY MERIDIANS

We have already mentioned the meridians which run in a "centrifugal" and "centripetal" direction all over the body, with their starting points or ends at the extremities. According to the traditional view, these vertical meridians are not only interlinked at their ends by "connecting bridges." There are also other tiny links between them; these run in a horizontal direction and connect the individual meridians. Traditional medical science calls such links *Lo,* or "threads."

If we regard the main meridians as rivers within the "macrocosmic and microcosmic" framework of the universe, then we can grade these *Lo* links as tributaries or brooks, some of which flow into other "rivers" and thus form transverse links between the "rivers." If, by a similar analogy, we regard the main meridians as "highways," then the *Lo* links can be taken as "byways."[83]

Because of this, the existence of the subsidiary meridians is closely bound up with the function of the *Lo* links. In addition to the main and special meridians there is in fact a further "circulation network," consisting of a process of change whereby one section of a meridian connects with another meridian by means of a *Lo* link and thus acts as a meridian on its own account. In such cases a *Yang* meridian is always connected to a *Yin* meridian, and vice versa.

These so-called subordinate meridians begin at the knee or the elbow, skirt the trunk, and join up again with another meridian at a certain point.

Thus there are the following subordinate meridians:

1. Bladder meridian (*Yang*) + kidney meridian (*Yin*)
2. Gall bladder meridian (*Yang*) + liver meridian (*Yin*)
3. Stomach meridian (*Yang*) + spleen meridian (*Yin*)
4. Small intestine meridian (*Yang*) + heart meridian (*Yin*)
5. "Triple warmer" meridian (*Yang*) + circulation meridian (*Yin*)
6. Large intestine meridian (*Yang*) + lung meridian (*Yin*).[84]

Up till now the workings of the subordinate meridians have been determined exclusively on an empirical basis. Their value is seen to lie in a subtle harmonization of organic function and vegetative equilibrium. There is frequent reference to them in the relevant works by modern Chinese authors,[85] but Chu Lien does not discuss them in her book, and Western authors also ignore them.

THE MUSCULAR MERIDIANS

The traditional art of healing also refers to meridians which—primarily, at least—are not connected to the inner organs but affect the functions of the skin and muscles.

In accordance with the "ruling" *Yin-Yang* principle these meridians, too, are divided into *Yin* and *Yang*. These are the twelve muscular meridians, whose body points are already included on the twelve main meridians. This new classification is essentially based on their potential ability to affect skin and muscular ailments, and clearly bears out the theory that the

73

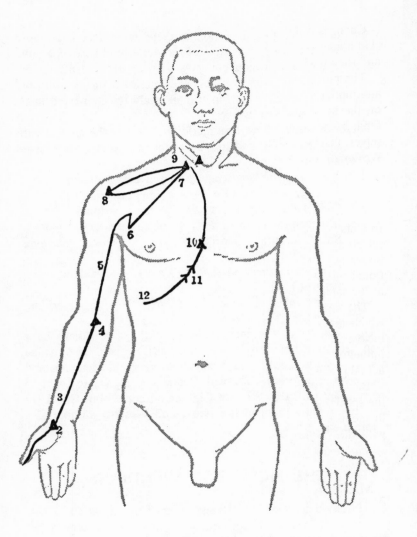

FIGURE 19
THE MUSCULAR MERIDIAN BELONGING TO THE LUNG MERIDIANS
(For an explanation of symbols see Figure 5.)

stimulation points of the body were the first to be discovered, and that the links between them, the meridians, were determined later.

Changes in the muscular meridians are associated either with skin ailments, such as rashes or eczema, or with muscular cramp and rheumatic pains.

The muscular meridians are frequently mentioned both in old and modern traditional medical books. Chu Lien uses the points on the muscular meridians when referring to treatment of this kind, but does not go into any detail about the meridians themselves. There are no references at all to such meridians in Western publications.[86]

THE SPECIAL POINTS

In Chinese works on the subject the *Lo* or connecting points are referred to as "special points" of the body. Modern Chinese books list fifteen such points and give their location and operational interconnection.[87] Each of these special points functions at the same time as a point within the framework of a meridian.

The special points can lie between two adjacent meridians which are under the influence of the same element, but which have a different *Yin-Yang* character; they exercise a harmonizing influence, and have consequently proved particularly effective in actual practice.

Bachmann is among the European authors who take note of the special points. He follows Ferreyrolles and Soulié de Morant in mentioning 31 points of the body which are not connected with the system of meridians. He also describes 20 additional *special points* which belong to one of the main meridians.[88]

MERIDIANS AND ACUPUNCTURE POINTS IN THE LIGHT OF MODERN RESEARCH

Western medical science has evaluated the points on the body and the meridians linking them in various ways. Some doctors have considered the whole thing to be quackery and regard the Chinese art of healing, both in theory and in practice, as an outmoded, unscientific system. Other scientists are of the opinion that this system of meridians and body points is a valuable one, despite the old-fashioned nomenclature, and seek to relate it to

75

certain sections or functional cycles of the circulatory and nervous systems. Hübotter,[89] for example, relates the *Yin* meridians to the arteries and the *Yang* meridians, on the other hand, to the nerve pathways. He associates, for instance, the lung meridian with the radial, axial, and subclavian arteries, and the large intestine meridian, on the other hand, with the branches of the radial nerve. The Japanese Ishikawa, and the Frenchmen Ribet and Nessler,[90] come to similar conclusions. These comparisons, however, are inadequate, since they do not provide a complete explanation, and instead of coming to any decision as to the value of the Chinese medical heritage, merely lose themselves in a mass of detail.

The existence of the meridians and points on the body, often regarded as mythical, can in fact be proved by experiment. In China and the Soviet Union, and also in Europe, highly sensitive electropotentiometers have been developed for measuring skin resistance. These have recorded constant potential values along the meridians but fluctuating ones elsewhere.

Similar recordings have been made in Germany by R. Voll-Plochingen, using his "electro-acupuncture" device. Two special instruments were designed in the biophysical institute of the Lomonosow University in Moscow precisely for locating such points on the body. On one of these electronic instruments an electrode illuminates a control light as soon as it makes contact with a body point. The second device, a portable one, produces acoustic signals when the skin is rubbed; the signals are clearly weaker at the body points. Both instruments confirm the supposition that the points are located in the connective tissue. It has also been proved that the electric potential of skin resistance on and near the body is of various quality. The measurements have likewise confirmed that the connective tissue is looser in the vicinity of the points.

The principle behind the Soviet "acoustic" instrument is based on the same finding. The sound produced by rubbing the skin is reproduced in varying degrees of strength by the media. The weaker sound denotes looser connective tissue and thus determines the points that are being looked for.[91]

A constant skin resistance can be recorded at all the points along a meridian; this is even possible on corpses.[92]

Durville and Bisky have published the results of various electrophysical skin resistance measurements. They have located some 400 points on the head alone, the positions of which could all be precisely determined; in most cases they coincide with the points already known from the Chinese art of healing.[93]

Various publications of Chinese doctors who have had modern training, and also European works on the subject, are agreed that the presence of the meridians and body points is associated with the sensitivity of the autonomic nervous system, that is, the peripheral nervous system which supplies the organs involved in self-preservation, growth, and reproduction—in other words, with the internal (visceral) organs, all glands, the smooth musculature, the myocardial musculature, the skin, and the mucous membrane. European medicine also considers it probable that the striated musculature, too, is to a certain extent autonomically innervated. The autonomic nervous system is also closely associated with the endocrine glands.

The autonomic nervous system is, however, closely linked not only to the internal organs but also to the "center," consisting of the brain and the spinal cord. It regulates and coordinates the vital processes of the whole organism, such as respiration, digestion, metabolism, the maintenance of the correct degree of heat and water content in the body, and, to a certain extent, reproduction as well. The basic phenomena of the neurobiological processes which occur in the autonomic nervous system are the so-called visceral reflexes. There is an essential difference between these and the biological purpose of the so-called somatic reflexes of the brain and spinal column. Whereas the somatic reflexes control the relationship of the whole organism to its environment, the task of the visceral reflexes is to maintain the dynamic equilibrium of the biological processes and ensure that the organs function harmoniously together.

The autonomic nervous system is divided—depending on the section of the central nervous system from which the preganglionic nerve cords emanate—into the sympathetic and the parasympathetic nervous systems. Both systems react in conflicting ways (antagonistically) to medicaments and chemicals. Almost all internal organs are innervated sympathetically and parasympathetically.[94]

77

Stimulation of the meridians and points of the body affects the autonomic nervous system, as explained above, and helps the organs to function harmoniously. This applies in particular to acupuncture and moxibustion, both of which will be described later, and also to the effects of remedial massage.

Let us now quote from some modern views. According to W. Lang, the meridians are not nerve pathways in the area of the skin, but central connecting links in the spinal cord and brain stem, which radiate to the periphery.[95] Lang also mentions the connection between the spinal cord segments and the meridians. In view of the fact that the segmental system is arranged horizontally, whereas the meridians run vertically, he concludes that

---

FIGURE 20

(From the work by Chu Lien; the original diagram is in color.)
Explanation of symbols:

A. preganglionic fibers of the sympathetic nerve
B. ganglia of the sympathetic nerve
C. postganglionic fibers of the sympathetic nerve
D. preganglionic fibers of the parasympathetic nerve
E. ganglia of the parasympathetic nerve
F. postganglionic fibers of the parasympathetic nerve.

The significance of the Chinese lettering beside the various numbers is as follows:

1. cerebrum
2. between-brain
3. mid-brain
4. cerebellum
5. medulla oblongata
6. cervical spinal cord segments
7. thoracic spinal cord segments
8. vasomotors of the skin and sweat glands
9. lumbar spinal cord segments
10. sacral spinal cord segments
11. pelvic nerve
12. pelvic ganglion
13. lower mesenteric ganglion
14. splanchnic nerves
15. upper mesenteric ganglion
16. intestinal ganglion
17. large nerves of internal organs
18. sympathetic artery
19. vagus nerve
20. tympanic nerve
21. oculomotor nerve.

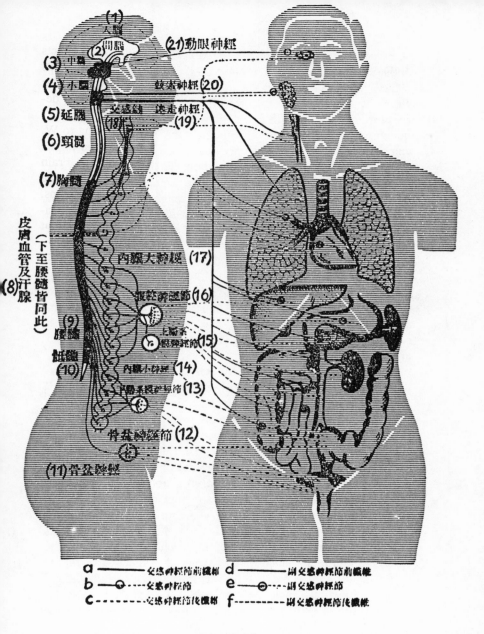

FIGURE 20

THE ASSOCIATED AREAS OF THE AUTONOMIC NERVOUS SYSTEM

79

the efficacy of acupuncture and moxibustion depends not only on the individual segments but also on their "interconnection."[96]

Lang has also examined the extension of the stimulation produced by acupuncture and moxibustion, beginning with the receptor zone on the skin and ending in the appropriate area of the cortex. According to his findings the peripheral neurite, which is rooted in the receptor area of the skin, runs to the spinal ganglion and conveys stimulation via the central neurites to the first synapse of the appropriate segment of the spinal cord. Here the second neuron begins through which stimulation reaches the thalamus as far as the second synapse. Finally, the third neuron conveys stimulation to the appropriate area of the cortex.[97]

Lang reports on an experiment during which he stimulated the *Ho-ku* point on a patient (this point is located on the hand, where the first and second wrist bones meet). The patient also experienced stimulation on the underarm, on the upper arm, and in the region of the neck and nose. This stimulus path corresponds to the large intestine meridian of the traditional art of healing.

Lang explained this result by stating that the nerve fibers, although isolated, are "open" at the synapses, or "relay points." It was here that there would thus be a link with the connecting cells and fibers of the extrapyramidal system, which would produce the above-mentioned phenomena.[98]

According to the Japanese scientist Fujita, the responsiveness of the points of the body is due not only to the vasoneural links but also to the musculature, the humoral-physiological changes in which would also be apparent on the periphery.[99] The stimulus affects not only the skin but the musculature as well. According to Fujita, the extensors and the hollow organs with a smooth musculature are *Yang* in character, whereas the flexors and the so-called parenchymatous organs are *Yin*.[100]

Bachmann's view is that the central, sensory, and visceral areas of function should be regarded as one unified whole together with the periphery, and it is to this that he attributes the efficacy of stimulation therapy.[101]

The views of modern acupuncture researchers are therefore at variance, and the methods by which the meridians and the points on the body work have still not been convincingly explained. According to Professor Huard, their explanation is a problem of physiology, not morphology. He notes that the Oriental (that is, Chinese and Soviet) interpreters generally take Pavlov's nervism as a starting point and proceed from there.[102] Let us therefore examine the basic essentials of this theory.

Even before Pavlov (1849–1936) began his research, it was known that the brain was a vital organ, but neither psychology nor physiology could supply a scientifically satisfactory explanation of its function, that is, of the biological processes which occurred in it. It is to Pavlov's credit that he sought to explain the basic biological processes of higher nervous activity in an objective way, namely, by means of biological experiments. He was able to show that the basic phenomena of higher nervous activity were specific reflex processes of the cerebral cortex. By means of experiments on animals—mainly dogs—he discovered that various stimuli, not associated with any particular conditions (such as food), caused a reflex action which he called an "unconditioned reflex."

Sound, or the sight of the keeper, or other stimuli which could affect the animal's behavior and indeed setting its unconditioned reflexes into motion were referred to by Pavlov as "conditioned stimuli," and the reflex action which they initiated he called a "conditioned reflex."[103] He also pointed out that opposing or excessive stimuli in the cerebral cortex caused inhibitions to develop and that these affected the entire nervous system and, through it, the whole organism. The reaction against excessive stimulation is called defensive inhibition.

The cerebral cortex is linked not only to the musculature and the sense organs but also, via neural connections, to the internal organs, so that the reflexes can affect the functioning of the latter as well. The cerebral cortex thus influences the activity of all organs and controls organic and somatic functions.

Thus Pavlov's "nervism" does not merely regard only the organism as a whole; it takes into account the indissoluble interrelationship between organism and environment. We shall now determine how meridians and acupuncture points can be assessed on the basis of Pavlovian theory.

According to Chu Lien,[104] the stimuli which affect individual

81

points on the body produce reactions throughout the entire nervous system as well as in the cerebral cortex. Mild stimuli have a tonifying effect, whereas strong ones can engender a so-called defensive inhibition, which was used for sedation purposes in the traditional art of healing. Chu Lien associates the reactions caused by acupuncture and moxibustion with the function of the cerebral cortex. There is a comprehensive division of function and organization among the cells of the body, covering digestion, respiration, metabolism, circulation, the locomotor system, and internal secretion, all of which are controlled by the nervous system.

The cerebral cortex coordinates and controls all functional processes at the highest level, thus making the body a unified whole.[105] A similar view is expressed by Wang Hsüeh-tai, who regards the traditional methods of healing, particularly acupuncture and moxibustion, as stimulation therapy.[106]

The Soviet researchers share the views of their Chinese colleagues. W. G. Wogralik, I. M. Goldberg, and N. J. Ingamdschanov refer to treatment carried out on meridians and points on the body as "stimulation therapy" or "reflex therapy." W. P. Filatov attributes successful cures achieved by acupuncture and moxibustion to biological stimulation.[107]

Although opinions are still at variance regarding the explanation of the traditional Chinese art of healing, practical experience has shown that the procedures are basically sound. In certain individual cases the traditional Chinese methods produce even better results than modern therapy.

We have previously noted that several Far Eastern countries have in recent years been conducting research into traditional Chinese medicine in the light of modern science. Among these is North Korea, where studies of the meridian system have led to important discoveries in the fields of microscopic anatomy and histology, and in other branches of science as well.

On November 30, 1963, the research findings of the Meridian Research Center in North Korea, under the direction of biology professor Kim Bong Han, were published in the capital of Pyongyang. Professor Kim Bong Han reported on his pioneering discoveries in the presence of a number of leading figures in the field of science. His work, together with relevant documents, was dispatched to academies of science all over the world. In the appendix to this book we have reproduced the table of contents of this extraordinarily important study as published in the December 14, 1963, edition of the newspaper *Renmin Ribao*. The paper entitled "On the Meridian System" describes this system in detail, together with its morphological, experimental-physiological, biochemical, histochemical, and bioelectric implications.

The international gathering of scientists in Pyongyang decided to call the structure of traditional acupuncture points discovered by Kim Bong Han "Bonghan corpuscles" (*corpusculum Bong-hani*), the tube-like connective structure of the corpuscles "Bonghan ducts" (*ductus Bonghani*), and the liquid circulating in it "Bonghan fluid" (*liquor Bonghani*).

The "Bonghan corpuscles" are found not only in the reticular layer of the skin but also in the deep layer of the connective tissue, in the vicinity of the blood and lymphatic vessels and even in the area of the internal organs; they are therefore divided into "surface" and "deep layer" Bonghan corpuscles. All of these corpuscles are interconnected by tube-like structures. These tubes run along the blood vessels, but outside them, and are interconnected. They are called "Bonghan ducts outside the blood vessels" in contrast to the "floating ducts" in the blood vessels and lymphatic vessels. Each of these "floating ducts" can connect with the above-mentioned "Bonghan corpuscles." This discovery poses new problems in the field of anatomical histology.

It was possible to prove this circulation in the tubes by several methods—for example, by radioactive means, using a P 32 phosphorus isotope, together with autoradiography. The phosphorus injected into the corpuscles of the surface layer penetrated the "Bonghan ducts" of the surface layer in the same way as did the phosphorus injected into the deep layer corpuscles, thus demonstrating the circulation of the "Bonghan fluid."

The meridian system has other definite bioelectric features. The bioelectric currents discharged from the various "Bonghan corpuscles" in the course of experiments differ from each other as regards wave group, frequency, and amplitude of oscillation.

83

Similarly, there are three types of ascertainable changes of electric potential in the waves, namely, periodically alternating, unidirectional, and unattenuated waves. The experiments also showed that the stimuli induced by the effect of various medicaments are also traceable in bioelectric changes in the "Bonghan corpuscles." The discovery of bioelectric characteristics of this kind made it possible to investigate the connections between the points on the body and certain internal organs associated with them. The bioelectric conductivity of the entire meridian system can similarly be proved.

Just as important are the results of the biochemical and histological investigations. The quantitative phosphorus analysis of the liquid in the "Bonghan corpuscles" and in the "Bonghan ducts" proved the presence of desoxyribonucleic acid and ribonucleic acid. At the same time, it was also discovered that the so-called "Bonghan fluid" has no cells, but merely contains a large number of basophile substances. This sounds very odd, since experts know that DNA (desoxyribonucleic acid) occurs only in the cell nucleus, whereas RNA (ribonucleic acid) appears only in the cytoplasm. These discoveries open up the way for new research and investigation, for the questions they raise affect basic biological problems, such as heredity, cell division, functions and proteometabolism, and so on.

This short description may serve to show the extraordinary importance of the results of research in Korea. There is no doubt that, once international control checks are completed, the discoveries of Professor Kim Bong Han and his colleagues will not only mark an important step forward in the development of medical knowledge, but will also bring the traditional Chinese art of healing closer to modern medical science.

FEELING THE PULSE

Feeling the pulse occupies a position of special importance in Chinese medicine. We have already noted that knowledge of this subject extends back to the 5th century B.C. According to tradition, it was the great Chinese doctor of antique times, Pien Ch'üeh, who first carried out diagnoses by means of the pulse.

All old medical works devote much space to the varying qualities of the pulse; both the "Su-Wên"[108] and the "Ling Shu"[109] contain several sections on the subject. The *Book of Ailments*, attributed to Pien Ch'üeh although it was probably not written until the Han dynasty, and the famous treatise by Wang Shu-he entitled the *Book of the Pulse* (*Mai Ching*) are both epoch-making in this particular field. Mention must also be made of the well-known work compiled by the 16th-century doctor and pharmacologist Li Shih-chên, *The Eight Special Meridians;* this book also deals in detail with the examination of the pulse, and the categories laid down therein are still used today by doctors who have been trained in the traditional way.

What exactly is meant by the pulse?

Modern medicine defines it as the rhythmic pulsation which can be detected either by instruments or by laying the point of one finger on the arteries. The blood pumped out of the left ventricle distends the wall of the aorta. This rhythmical expansion is transmitted in waves along the flexible sides of the arteries by means of the onrush of blood, thus causing the pulsation of the vascular walls. Normal procedure in the West is to take the pulse by feeling the radial artery (*arteria radialis*). The pulse provides information about the rhythm and frequency of the heartbeats and about the condition of the aortic valves.[110]

Chinese doctors take the pulse by feeling not only the radial artery referred to above but the arteries of the neck and legs as well. Chinese medicine constructed an entire diagnostic system by means of feeling the pulse on the *arteria radialis*. This method is based on the idea that, by merely feeling the pulse, a doctor can determine not only the condition of the heart and the aortic valves, but also whether the internal organs referred to as *Tsang* and *Fu* are in good or bad order. The pulse is taken on the *arteria radialis* of both forearms, the doctor placing three fingers on each radial artery and exerting varying degrees of pressure.

Gentle pressure reveals the condition of the so-called *Yang* organs, otherwise known as the *Fu's* or active organs. By exerting heavier pressure down to the "deep level" it is possible to determine the state of the *Yin* organs, otherwise known as the *Tsang's* or storage organs. By feeling the three relevant places

85

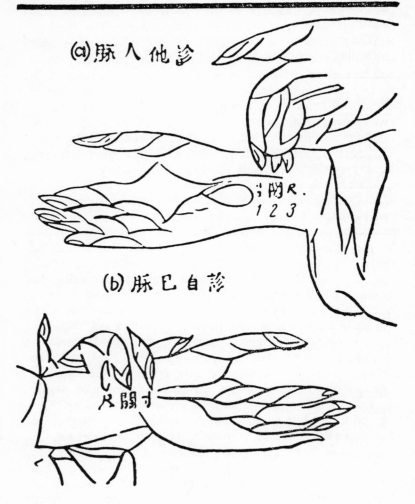

FIGURE 21
METHODS OF FEELING THE PULSE
(From *Compendium of Acupuncture and Moxibustion*, Ming period.)
A. Feeling another person's pulse.
B. Feeling one's own pulse.
(The Chinese characters and figures denote in each case the point where
the pulse is felt.)

86

on the *arteria radialis* of the left and right forearms the doctor can also determine the condition of each of the three *Yang* and *Yin* organs.

The condition of the following meridians can be determined by feeling the pulse:

On left arteria radials	By exerting slight pressure	By exerting strong pressure
With point of index finger	small intestine	heart
With point of middle finger	gall bladder	liver
With point of third finger	urinary bladder	kidneys
On right arteria radialis	By exerting slight pressure	By exerting strong pressure
With point of index finger	large intestine	lungs
With point of middle finger	stomach	spleen
With point of third finger	"triple warmer"	"controller of the heart"

It is possible, of course, to detect a wide range of variations. Both methods of feeling the pulse enable the doctor to determine whether it is "large" or "wiry" (*Yin* or *Yang* condition), reflecting either a balanced or disturbed rhythm and denoting the frequency and arterial pressure. The book entitled *A Summary of the Traditional Chinese Art of Healing* mentions 28 grades of pulse together with their characteristics and the bodily ailments revealed by each specific type.[111]

The problem of feeling the pulse is closely linked to tonification and sedation. Those doctors who remain true to tradition maintain from their own experience that the tonification of a meridian which applies to an organ belonging to the *arteria radialis* on the left forearm has a sedative effect on a meridian belonging to the same pulse point on the right forearm, and vice versa. This can be shown as follows:

Right arteria radialis	Left arteria radialis
small intestine	large intestine
heart	lungs
gall bladder	stomach
liver	spleen
urinary bladder	"triple warmer"
kidneys	"controller of the heart"

According to this rule, stimulation of the point of tonification on the liver meridian, for example, would have a sedative effect in the region of the spleen meridian; stimulation of the sedation point on the spleen meridian, on the other hand, would tonify the liver meridian.[112]

Modern doctors have doubts about this traditional technique of feeling the pulse, because the method is based on highly subjective assumptions. Nevertheless, there are thousands of years of experience to support it, and investigations carried out jointly by French doctors and their Chinese colleagues of the old traditional school have provided concrete proof of its efficacy. In 79 per cent of the test cases the diagnoses coincided, although the Chinese doctors made theirs merely by feeling the pulse.[113]

According to the Japanese scientist Fujita, variations in the pulse beat on the *arteria radialis* can indicate irregularities in the functioning of various organs. According to Bachmann, the superficially felt pulse relates to the dilation of the artery wall, whereas the deep pulse applies to blood pressure. The former would correspond to the previously mentioned hollow organs, which consist of smooth muscular fibers, that is to say, the *Yang* organs, whereas the latter, by virtue of its close association with the blood circulation, would correspond to the so-called *Yin* organs.[114] Stiefvater also considers the so-called peripheral pulse to be of value for diagnostic purposes. Chinese physicians have long been aware of it, and are of the opinion that this pulse, too, may indicate irregularities in the functioning of certain organs. Stiefvater's explanation is that the peripheral pulses are located at points where the arteries are relatively close to the skin surface (as on the head, neck, arms, knuckles), while the arteries in turn are associated anatomically with the internal organs.[115]

Although modern medicine regards the recognition of such various pulse qualities as being uncertain and too dependent on subjective impulses, it should be noted that the ability to detect such differences depends to a large extent on the more delicate sense of touch possessed by Orientals. It can, however, also be partly explained away by the fact that the passing on of the traditional medical experience from father to son generally began when the child was at a very early age, so that the development of the sense of touch proceeded contemporaneously with the general training of the future doctor. It goes without saying that a great deal of research requires to be done on this aspect of Chinese medicine.

CAUSES OF ILLNESS

According to the traditional art of healing, the causes of illness are divided into nine groups, namely: [116]

1. The six "bad" causes: wind, cold, heat, damp, dryness, and fire
2. the epidemics
3. the seven emotional states: joy, anger, anxiety, worry, grief, fear, and shock
4. physical upsets and states of exhaustion caused by various foodstuffs and beverages
5. excessive sexual activity
6. injuries, including bites from snakes and rabid animals
7. visceral parasites
8. poisoning, including poisonous drugs
9. hereditary factors.

Let us consider each of these causes in turn.

The physical upsets brought about by the *six "bad" causes* have already been referred to in our chapter "Man and Climate." These are brought on largely by the effects of the seasons on the organism. We noted, for example, that illnesses caused by the wind generally occur more frequently in spring and that they represent, from the medical point of view, the result of inadequate heat control. The "Su-Wên" goes into great detail on the subject of the effects of windy weather on the organism, and lists among the specific ailments "catarrh," "coughing," "stuffed-up nose," and "headaches." The wind is referred to as the "cause of a hundredfold illnesses."[117]

Cold takes effect mainly in winter, when arthritic complaints, colic, and diarrhea may occur.[118] Heat, that is to say, in summer, is associated with headaches, fits of sweating, and circulatory disorders. Damp, which coincides with late summer in

89

China, can cause boils, jaundice, and arthritis. The illnesses caused by dryness—whether dry heat or dry cold—occur mainly in autumn, and are associated with headaches, coughing, vomiting, sore throat, or "stabbing pains" in the chest. And, finally, fire causes inflammation, reddening, and tumors.

This list contains symptoms rather than actual illnesses. Moreover, association of the six "bad" causes with the seasons indicates an attempt to reduce the general Chinese experience and the various regional theories to a common denominator.

The *various epidemics* are dealt with even in the very oldest medical works, revealing what was for those early days a remarkable understanding of cause and effect. Thus we find accounts showing that epidemics can be spread by people, animals (particularly rats), foul water, polluted air, and human breath. One result of such knowledge, incidentally, was the consumption of so much boiled tea and water.

Cholera, plague, diphtheria, and smallpox are often given as examples of epidemics. In the fight against smallpox China discovered what is called natural immunity and was the first country in the world to exploit it. This immunization was achieved by "vaccinating" healthy people with secretions from the vesicles of smallpox sufferers. The normally milder infection which followed the "vaccination" produced life-long immunity. Such "protective vaccination" as we have already noted, was carried out by having the patient sniff some dried secretion from smallpox vesicles up his nose, or by rubbing it into the mucous membrane. This procedure, though known in China since time immemorial, did not, however, become generally widespread until the 16th century.[119]

An imbalance in any of the seven *emotional states,* according to traditional medical science, can also cause physical disturbance. Strangely enough, joy is included among the unbalanced emotions—that is to say, sudden, overwhelming joy, when "the rejoicing person's soul is surprised and laid bare, instead of remaining concealed."[120] In other words, when someone is so overjoyed that he "loses his reason." Intense anger produces rushes of blood and can cause disorders of the liver. Over-anxiety can affect the lungs. Worry and imagination are said to upset the functioning of the spleen. Grief and sadness can cause heart disease.[121] Fear and shock can lead to serious circulatory disorders.[122] Fear differs from shock inasmuch as the person concerned knows the reason for his fear but does not know in advance the causes of his shock.

The disorders caused by the various emotional states are not merely considered in conjunction with empirical experiences; an attempt is made to link them to theory, although the philosophical approach may be outmoded. Nevertheless, the fact is worth noting that, even at that early date, Chinese medicine was aware of psychophysical interrelationships and recognized the importance of psychic factors as a cause of physical disorders.[123]

Disorders caused by foodstuffs and beverages are due to bad food and excessive eating and drinking. The results include stomach upsets, digestive disorders, constipation, and, in the case of over-indulgence in alcohol, delirium. The traditional art of healing which has been handed down also associates the five qualities of taste with physical disorders.

Exhaustion can also occur in conjunction with irregular breathing, sweating, and cardiac complaints. It can result from the constant straining of the organism as a whole, or of individual organs. According to the "Su-Wên,"[124] "prolonged staring affects the blood, prolonged standing harms the bones, and lengthy walking wearies the muscles."

Excessive sexual activity can also produce physical disorders. The "Ling Shu"[125] states that "kidney trouble may result from excessive sexual appetite." A balanced sex life is closely bound up with harmony of the internal organs and the whole body. Outward signs of a well-balanced sexuality are "cleanliness of face and skin," a "clear glance," and "keenness of hearing." Sexual excesses can, in the long run, cause irregular menstruation among women and, in the case of men, lead to fever, cardiac complaints, sacralgia, cold hands and feet, and impotence or premature ejaculation of semen.[126]

Under the heading *"injuries, including bites from snakes and rabid animals,"* Chinese medicine lists wounds from stabbing and shooting, broken bones, sprains, snake bites (which occur fairly often in South China), and bites from rabid animals.[127]

The traditional art of healing recognizes several types of

91

visceral parasites, including, among others, the worms known as *Hui-ch'ung, Jao-ch'ung,* and *Ts'un-pai-ch'ung.* The *Hui-ch'ung* is described as follows: "it is normally a foot long, although there are some which are 5 to 6 inches long; whenever it begins to move, the patient feels abdominal pains." The helminth referred to as *Jao-ch'ung* "is quite small and shaped like a caterpillar." The *Ts'un-pai-ch'ung* "grows to about an inch in length; it is white in color, small and narrow, sets the *Tsang's* and *Fu's* in motion, and weakens them."[128] It is probable that the *Hui-ch'ung* can be equated with the *Taenia solium* and the *Jao-ch'ung* with the *Taenia echinococcus* (types of tapeworm), whereas the *Ts'un-pai-ch'ung* is presumably the female of the threadworm (*Enterobius vermicularis*).

In this connection an age-old superstition is worth mentioning. In ancient China there was a certain worm which was used for bewitching people. It was called *Ku* and it can be assumed that it was a helminth. It was employed in conjunction with magic rites and incantations. A handful of worms were put into a receptacle and the magic ingredients were added. The receptacle was then covered up and allowed to remain untouched for a year. The worms inside were soon starving and ate one another up, the last survivor being the *Ku*. This worm was especially suitable for casting a spell since, according to superstition, it now had concentrated all the "poison" contained in those it had eaten up. It was used to "destroy" unpopular people whom one wanted to get rid of. It is no longer possible to determine whether, and how, it was successful, but the *Ku* worm was in any event surrounded by an aura of superstition.

Poisoning can be caused by foodstuffs, particularly bad fish or meat—certainly no rare occurrence in view of the Chinese climate. Drugs and plants, however, can also have a toxic effect, as, for example, the *Pa-t'ou* (*Croton tiglium*), from the seed of which croton oil is obtained, the *Wu-t'ou* (*Aconitum chinense* or Chinese aconite), and others. Medicaments of inorganic origin, too, such as the minerals sulphur and arsenic, which have been known since time immemorial, can produce poisonous effects.[129]

Finally, as far as *hereditary factors* are concerned, the old works on the subject state that, at conception, *Ching* (sperm and ovum) and *Ch'i* (energy) unite and transmit the characteristics of the parents to the child.[130] Traditional medicine is also concerned with the inheritance of diseases. In the book attributed to him the Yellow Emperor asks his minister and court physician, Ch'i Po: ". . . a person is born who is epileptic. How is his illness explained and where did he get it from?" To this Ch'i Po answers: "This illness is known as the 'affliction of the maternal womb.' The fetus was stricken when the mother received a sudden shock while it was still in her body. The *Ch'i* (energy) increased, but did not decrease again, so that it was unable to unite with the *Ching* (sperm and ovum); that is why the child you are referring to became an epileptic."[131]

The case described above represents, it is true, pre-natal injury rather than an actual "inheritance," but Chinese medical scientists can also quote specific examples where physical characteristics have been transmitted from parents to children.

TRADITIONAL DIAGNOSES AND TREATMENT

Doctors trained in the traditional school arrive at their diagnoses by means of the so-called "eight principles" and the "four methods of examination." In accordance with the eight principles, the first thing to be done is to ascertain whether the illness is *Yin* or *Yang* in character, whether it has external or internal symptoms, whether it is of a cold or warm nature, and finally whether it is due to an increased or reduced function.

The four methods of examination consist of looking, listening, questioning, and feeling the pulse.

The use of the *Yin-Yang* principle in arriving at a diagnosis reveals a link between philosophy and practice. Yin is associated with an "internal," "cold," and reduced function, while *Yang,* on the other hand, is associated with an "external," "warm," and increased function. "In the case of *Yang* illnesses the patient will not lie still; he is lively and talkative; his breath comes in sporadic gasps; he requires to be cooled down; and in

93

addition he is constantly thirsty and his pulse is accelerated."

"A patient suffering from a *Yin* illness is limp; he does not wish to see anyone; he will not talk; his body is cold, so that he requires warmth; his urine is milky and clouded; his pulse is weak and slow."[132]

As far as the *external* or *internal symptoms* are concerned, the eight "bad causes," to which reference has already been made, attack the "surface" of the body first. "The illness spreads from the surface of the skin along the meridians into the internal organs." The external or "cold" surface symptoms include headaches, inability to perspire, arthralgia, and a coated tongue. "Warm" surface symptoms include perspiration, thirst, and an accelerated pulse rate. Symptoms of "inner coldness" are a moist, coated tongue, absence of any feeling of thirst, vomiting, and diarrhea. Symptomatic of "inner heat" are a reddened tongue with a yellowish coating, thirst, and exhaustion. These symptoms can also be at variance with one another and may be both external and internal at one and the same time. Thus symptoms of "coldness" can appear on the "surface" together with others of "inner warmth" (for example, pains and limpness). Symptoms of "outer warmth" with "inner coldness" include, for example, headaches allied to fever and shivering. In arriving at diagnoses the traditional art of healing takes all possible combinations of symptoms into account. In the event of physical disorders the six *Yin* organs and the six *Yang* organs reveal increased or reduced functions, which, in turn, are either "cold" or "warm" and "external" or "internal" in nature. A doctor of the old school must therefore not only be able to recognize the individual symptoms with complete certainty; he must also be familiar with all the possible combinations in order to arrive at a correct diagnosis.[133] The aim and scope of this book do not permit a detailed description of all the symptoms.

Examination by looking, listening, questioning, and feeling the pulse is carried out as follows:

Examination by *looking* means that the doctor observes the patient's complexion, the color of his skin, together with his mouth, nose, tongue, eyes, teeth. Many conclusions can be drawn from the coating of the tongue in particular, and distinctions are made between "reddish, bluish, greenish, yellowish, greyish, and darkish coatings."

During *listening* the sound of the patient's breathing, together with his manner of coughing and speaking, are observed. This method of examination also includes observance of the patient's perspiration and the nature of his urine and stool.

Questioning enables the doctor to gain information about the patient's habits, background, and any circumstances which might affect his state of health. He also inquires about appetite, stool, and general health, and tries in this way to discover how much the patient knows about himself.[134]

Feeling the pulse, the last stage in the diagnosis, has already been discussed in detail in a previous section.

Once a diagnosis has been arrived at, the traditional doctors employ "lesser" or "greater" methods of treatment. "Lesser" methods include heat treatment or the prescription of emetics, laxatives, or diuretics. In the case of illnesses with "warm" symptoms, medicaments of a "cold" nature are administered, and vice versa. Sedatives are prescribed in order to reduce excessive organic activity, and strengthening medicaments for the treatment of hypofunction.

Included among the "greater" methods of treatment are acupuncture, moxibustion, respiratory therapy, remedial massage, physiotherapy, and, in certain cases, cupping as well. Respiratory therapy and physiotherapy are largely used for chronic illnesses.[135]

In addition to the various methods of remedial treatment, the *prevention* of illness is an old-age tradition in China. This becomes understandable when we consider the climate conditions in China. A correct balance between work, relaxation, and sleep and the "golden rules" of a moderate, "clean," and correct diet help to prevent illness. Diet, massage physiotherapy, sun bathing, and the use of water from hot springs can all have a preventative effect, and the rules for the prevention of infectious diseases and the methods recommended for proper adjustment to the weather and the seasons likewise apply here.

PART II

TRADITIONAL METHODS
OF TREATMENT

4

ACUPUNCTURE

In Part 1 we attempted to provide a survey of the principles and practice of the traditional art of healing in China. Essential to an understanding of traditional Chinese medicine is a thorough knowledge of its view on the relationship between Man and Nature, its acupuncture and meridian systems, and its detailed account of the causes and diagnoses of illness. We shall now consider acupuncture in greater detail—a subject, by the way, of much discussion today in Europe as well as in the Far East. A number of Western doctors are, in fact, engaged in elaborate investigations of this empiric art, for acupuncture has yielded a vast store of medical evidence which can provide even modern science with much valuable information.

As we have already noted, therapy by means of stimulation with a needle—under the Latinized name of *acupuncture* (from *acus*—needle, and *pungere*—to puncture)—has been practiced in China since early times. In the pre-Christian eras stone needles were used for this purpose. Later, presumably before the compilation of *The Yellow Emperor's Classic of Internal Medicine* (*Huang-ti Nei-ching*) metal needles were used instead.[136] This method of treatment consists basically of inserting one or more metal needles to varying depths at appropriate points of time. Treatment of this kind, either carried out once or repeated several times, is an aid to physical harmony and thus to the restoration of health.

Chinese and European writers alike tend to combine acupuncture with treatment by means of heating or burning (*moxi-*

99

bustion). This latter process consists basically of encouraging organic harmony by heating or burning those same points on the body which form the basis of acupuncture treatment. This will be dealt with more fully in the next chapter, but reference must be made here to a similar method on account of the sources concerned.

Of the roughly two to three hundred important Chinese works on this subject the following may be regarded as the most significant: the works entitled "Su-Wên" and "Ling Shu" from the collection known as *The Yellow Emperor's Classic of Internal Medicine (Huang-ti Nei-ching)*, the *Book of Ailments (Nan Ching)* from the Han period; *The First and Second Book (Chia-i Ching)* written by Huang-fu Mi during the Ch'in period; *A Thousand Ducat Prescriptions (Ch'ien Chin Fang)* of Sun Szû-miao from the Sui-T'ang period; the *Compendium of Acupuncture and Moxibustion (Chên-chiu Ta-ch'êng)* of Yang Chi-chou from the Ming period; and the collection entitled *The Golden Mirror of the Art of Healing (I-tsung Chin-chien)* dating from the 18th century A.D.

During the T'ang period acupuncture reached Japan and also spread into Korea and India. The first account of it to appear in Europe was in London in 1683, the author being the Dutch doctor Ten Rhyne. In 1712 Engelbrecht Kaempfer published a book entitled *Curatio Colicae per Acupuncturam Japonibus Usitata (The Curing of Diarrhea by means of Acupuncture as Used by the Japanese)*. Then follows an account of an unknown missionary in a book entitled *Description de l'Empire de la Chine et de la Tartarie Chinoise (Description of the Chinese Empire and Chinese Tartary)*, which appeared in Paris in 1735. In 1826 J. Cloquet compiled the first comprehensive account of acupuncture under the title *Traité de l'Acupuncture (A Treatise on Acupuncture)*.

All of these books, however, are to be regarded as curiosities rather than as serious scientific works. The first really significant treatise is P. Dabry's book, *La médicine chez les Chinois (Medicine Among the Chinese)*, which was published in Paris in 1863.

In the present century George Soulié de Morant—together with Ferreyrolles—compiled two critical accounts: *L'Acu-*

puncture en Chine et la Réflexothérapie Moderne (*Acupuncture in China and Modern Reflexotherapy*), which appeared in 1929, and *Les Aiguilles et les Moxas en Chine* (*Acupuncture and Moxibustion in China*), published in 1930. According to **P.** Huard, both accounts contain incorrect quotations.

Roger de la Fuye's excellent work, *Traité d'Acupuncture Chinoise sans Mystère* (*A Treatise on Chinese Acupuncture Shorn of Its Mystery*), which appeared in Paris in 1947, was followed in 1954 by A. Chamfrault's *Traité de Médicine Chinoise* (*A Treatise on Chinese Medicine*), published in Angoulême in 1954. The latter uses the Chinese sources referred to as "Su-Wên" and "Ling Shu," but unfortunately the rendering of these texts is neither accurate nor complete. Of the more important works written in French mention must finally be made of the significant and comprehensive book by Pierre Huard and Ming Wong entitled *La Médecine Chinoise au Cours des Siècles* (in English translation: *Chinese Medicine*), which gives a splendid summary of the history of the traditional art of healing, together with an account of the whole development of acupuncture. It is the most modern work on the history of Chinese medicine to have been published in the West.

A notable publication in German is Gerhard Bachmann's book entitled *Die Akupunktur, eine Ordnungstherapie* (*Acupuncture as Remedial Therapy*), Volumes I (text) and II (illustrations), published in Ulm/Danube in 1959. Also important are Erich Stiefvater's *Akupunktur als Neuraltherapie* (*Acupuncture as Neural Therapy*) (Ulm, 1956), and W. Lang's *Akupunktur und Nervensystem* (*Acupuncture and the Nervous System*) (Ulm, 1957), which summarized the results of neurological research with reference to acupuncture.

In the Soviet Union a Russian translation of Chu Lien's *Manual of Modern Acupuncture and Moxibustion* (*Hsin Chênchiu-hsüeh*) has appeared, together with works by W. G. Wogralik, Ingamdschanov, Boldirev, Korsakov, Krasnoselsky, Tükotschinskaja, and others and some 200 medical publications on relevant research results. In addition, a separate department of the Soviet Academy of Sciences is engaged on systematic research into acupuncture.

Among the countries of the Far West, Mongolia, Korea, Vietnam, India, and Japan are familiar with acupuncture and other Chinese methods of treatment. In Europe, acupuncture is not unknown in France, Germany, Austria, and Italy, and special publications devoted to the subject appear in France and Germany; these are the *Revue d'Acupuncture* and the *Deutsche Zeitschrift für Akupunktur*.

THE NEEDLES

In ancient times nine varying types of needles were used in China for acupuncture. Not all of them were, strictly speaking, needles; some were in the form of small lances, others had a ball point or a triple cutting edge. The latter were also used for opening tumors or for letting blood.

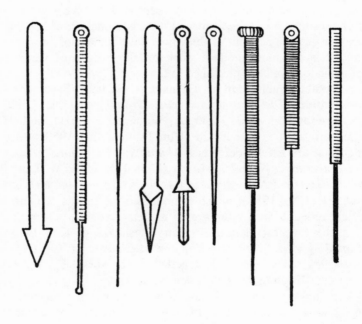

FIGURE 22
HISTORICAL ACUPUNCTURE NEEDLES
The nine different needles used in acupuncture in ancient times.

Nowadays *Hao-chên* needles with a triple cutting edge are used, together with so-called "skin needles." The needles comprise a holder and a stem. The "skin needle" has 5 to 6 separate adjacent needles combined in one holder; their points cover about about a square centimeter of skin. Generally speaking, the "skin needle" is used when treating small children, where it is merely a case of lightly tapping the appropriate points on the body.

The needles originally consisted of stone, but were later made of copper or iron. Nowadays gold, silver, and steel alloy needles are used for surgical instruments. As regards gold and silver

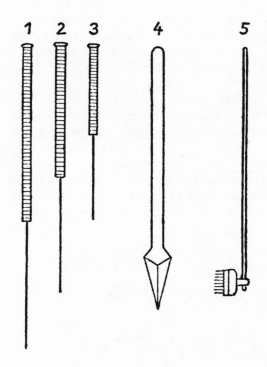

FIGURE 23
MODERN ACUPUNCTURE NEEDLES

Needles in use today: 1–3. *Hao-chên* needles (various lengths) 4. Triple-edged needle   5. Skin needle.

103

needles it is worth mentioning an interesting experiment carried out by Rumanian doctors, who were able to achieve varying physiological effects by using needles made of different materials. These Rumanian doctors—Prodescu, Stoicescu, and Bratu—experimented on dogs by puncturing the *Yüan* points of tonification on the gall bladder meridian. After a total of 120 experiments they ascertained that this produced an intensified secretion of bile, corresponding to the effect of a 20 per cent injection of decholin. In the case of gold needles the choleresis effect persisted, whereas with silver needles it gradually decreased.[137]

Doctors undergoing training first use small cotton pads on which to practice the angle of insertion, the amount of force to be used, and the correct way of holding the needle.

The acupuncture needles are disinfected before treatment commences—once they were dipped into an infusion of medicinal herbs; now they are boiled in the manner of hypodermic needles.

In China there is also what is called "natural acupuncture," whereby the patient "punctures" himself with one finger by pressing strongly on the appropriate acupuncture point. Almost every Chinese knows a certain number of important points on the body which can be treated in this way in cases of pain (toothache, headaches, spasmodic pains in the stomach) before a doctor is consulted. This type of treatment, however, falls rather within the sphere of Chinese remedial massage.

THREE BASIC QUESTIONS

The following three points must first of all be explained prior to the acupuncture itself:
1. the point of insertion and the appropriate bodily posture
2. direction and technique of the puncture
3. duration of puncture.

These basic questions are dealt with in detail both in old and modern Chinese works.[138]

Determining the Points of Insertion and Their Location on the Body

In the traditional art of healing the inch serves as the unit of measurement for purposes of locating the various acpuncture points. The tenth part of an inch (*Ts'un*) is called in Chinese *Fên*. Characteristic bone formations on the skeleton are used as reference points for measurement purposes. The Chinese inch, however, cannot be used as a standard measurement, since it does not cover all the constitutional differences between various patients. Thus an *individual* inch measurement applicable to all measurements taken on each patient's body was eventually created. This individual unit of measurement equals the length

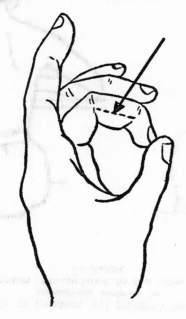

FIGURE 24
THE INDIVIDUAL "INCH" MEASUREMENT

The individual unit of measurement taken on the patient's middle finger, by means of which the location of, and distance between the various acupuncture points, can be determined.

105

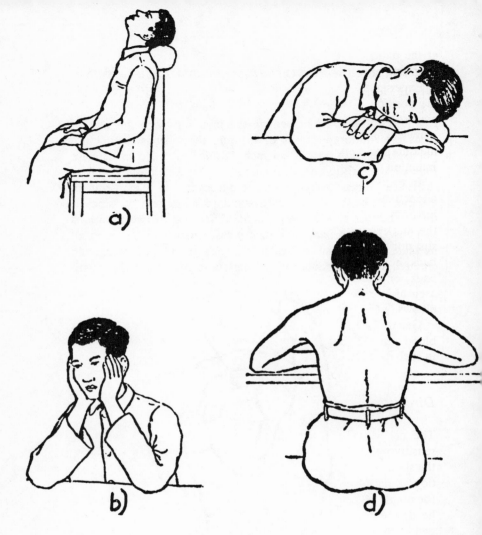

FIGURE 25
BODY POSTURES DURING ACUPUNCTURE, MOXIBUSTION,
OR MASSAGE TREATMENT

A. Head back and supported (for treatment of acupuncture points on the face)

B. Head supported on hands (for treatment of points on the forehead)

C. Head resting sideways (for treatment of points on one side of the face or on the ear or neck)

D. Sitting position, resting on the arms (for treatment of points on the back and neck).

106

of the patient's central phalanx on the middle finger, measured from one joint to the other.

Experienced doctors, however, only occasionally determine the position of acupuncture points by such a method; but beginners must make use of it in order to gain anatomical knowledge. Traditional doctors also have other methods of measurement for the head and the trunk, but it is not our intention to deal with these here.

In order that accurate puncture be assured, the patient must adopt a suitable posture. As a general rule the patient must prop his body firmly and not move, otherwise the needle will not hit the mark and may bend or even snap off. The patient usually sits during treatment and rests his forearms, on a table. His back, however, must also be supported. Lying on one's stomach, back, or side are also common positions. In the lying position a cushion is used for supporting the limbs, or as a pad for the elbows.

Generally speaking, points located in the vicinity of large blood vessels and near the eyes and ears should not be punctured; in such cases remedial massage or moxibustion is preferable.

Direction, Technique, and Duration of Acupuncture

The needle can be inserted at three main angles. The more sensitive points are stimulated at right angles to the surface of the skin, as are those located above thick layers of muscle. Insertion at an angle of 45° to the surface of the skin is used mostly for points on the chest, and at 12 to 15° for those on the face, head, and neck. The depth to which the needles are inserted depends on the location of the points. The normal depth of insertion ranges from 3 to 10 millimeters. Certain sources also mention depths of 6 to 7 inches, roughly equal to 12 to 14 centimeters.[139]

Insertion of the needle can be carried out in various ways. The doctor can, for example, press with his thumb on the skin near the point of insertion and then insert the needle alongside it. This procedure is usually adopted in the case of short needles.

With long needles, the so-called "guided insertion" method is used; using the thumb and index finger of his left hand, the doctor presses down the skin in the vicinity of the point of insertion in such a way that the point is located between the top sections of each finger. The needle is then guided down between the fingers. In this way it is comparatively easy to insert long needles as well, since the doctor can support his right hand, with which he holds the needle, on the back of his left one. There is thus less danger of the needle slipping or breaking. This technique is normally used on the small of the back, in the vicinity of the hips, and on the arms.

The needle can also be inserted into the small of the back and into the back itself if the doctor places his outstretched left hand on the patient in such a way that the selected point of insertion is located between the index and middle fingers.

For the face and head, and wherever the musculature is relatively thin, the doctor pinches the skin between two of his fingers and presses the needle down into the raised fold of skin towards the point of insertion.[140]

Since the correct point of insertion can easily be missed, the doctor normally fixes the localized point by exerting light pressure by means of the thumbnail.[141]

Acupuncture produces no sensations of pain, except on the fingers. The only sensations which may occasionally be felt are so-called synesthetic ones (a bitter or sour taste, numbness of the limbs, a feeling of warmth).

Insertion of the needle results in weak or strong stimuli being administered to the body, and acupuncture technique must take this into account. A weak stimulus normally has a tonifying effect, whereas a strong stimulus has a sedating one. Chu Lien explains this by suggesting that a short, weak stimulus (for example, in cases of general debility or hypofunction of the organs) causes increased activity of the organs because of its

---

FIGURE 26
A. Sitting upright with arms stretched forward
B. Lying sideways
C. Lying on the back with knees supported
D. Lying on the stomach with elbows propped.

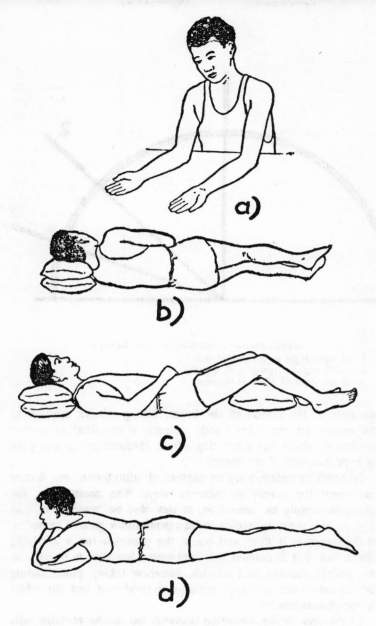

FIGURE 26
BODY POSTURES DURING ACUPUNCTURE, MOXIBUSTION,
OR MASSAGE TREATMENT

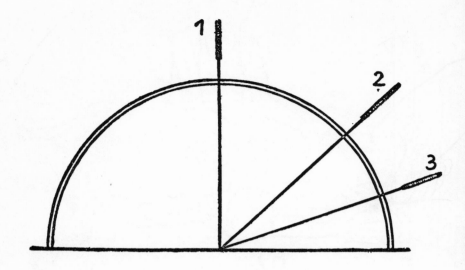

FIGURE 27
DIRECTION OF INSERTION OF THE NEEDLE
1. At right angle to surface of skin
2. At an angle of roughly 45 degrees
3. At an angle of 12 to 15 degrees.

reaction on the cortex of the brain. Strong stimuli applied to the cortex, on the other hand, generate a so-called *protective inhibition,* which has a sedating effect. (Indication: severe pain or hyperfunction of the organs.[142])

In order to obtain varying degrees of stimulation, the doctor can insert the needle in different ways. The needle can, for example, simply be jabbed in. It can also be "twirled in," as it were, in a rotating motion, which produces a greater stimulus. If the insertion is short and quick, the puncture has a tonifying effect, but if it is carried out intermittently—that is to say, as the patient exhales and inhales, insertion taking place during exhalation—then a strong stimulus is produced and the effect is one of sedation.[143]

In the case of a tonification stimulus the needle remains only briefly in the point of insertion. In the case of sedation, on the other hand, the needle is repeatedly raised and re-inserted more

110

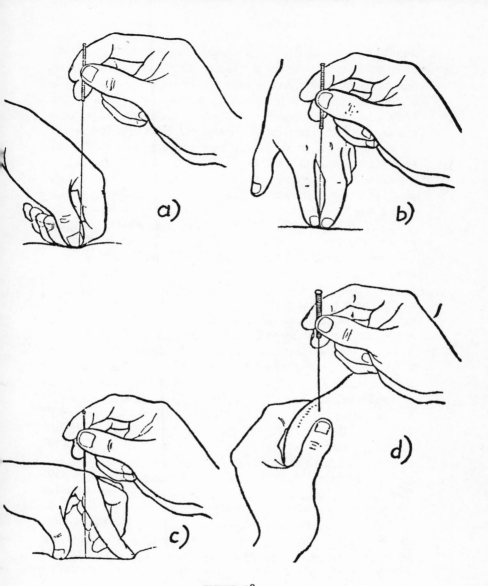

FIGURE 28
GUIDING THE ACUPUNCTURE NEEDLE
A. Insertion of long needle alongside thumbnail
B. Insertion of needle between two fingers
C. Insertion of needle into a taut fold on skin
D. Insertion of needle into a compressed fold on skin.

111

deeply, or even rotated in the point of insertion, in order to produce a stronger stimulus. This raising and re-inserting of the needle is also referred to as "bird-pecking." The length of time during which the needle is allowed to remain in the body can vary, depending on the persistence of the ailment and the patient's reaction; the needle can even remain inserted for several hours. In giving this treatment acupuncture doctors have also to bear in mind the individual patient's constitution, for there are some patients for whom relatively weak stimuli produce strong reactions, whereas in others even strong stimuli take a long time to attain the desired effect.

Physicians in ancient China followed complicated rules as regards the direction in which the needles should be rotated, the synchronization of the insertion of the needle with exhalation and inhalation, the period during which treatment should be given (day, season, position of the stars), and the nature of the ailment. Most of these rules are now nothing more than curiosities of medical history, although certain theories are worth checking on a systematic basis. Among these, for example, is the interconnection between the direction of rotation of the needle and the therapeutic effect. Chu Lien, who received modern medical training and is now doing research in the field of traditional medicine, has described these interconnections. In the treatment of facial convulsions (tics), for example, rotation of the needle in one particular direction did not produce any result at all, but when it was turned in the opposite direction the convulsions ceased at once. Chu Lien stresses the fact, however, that no general conclusions can be deduced from such an occurrence, since other cases did not produce comparable results.[144]

Chu Lien has also reported on the results of her further research into *Pu-hsieh* ("tonification-sedation"). Starting with the fact that tonification is based on weak stimulus, whereas sedation is associated with a protective inhibition of the cortex, she eventually concluded that the decisive factor as regards the effect of acupuncture treatment is the force with which the needle is inserted and not the direction in which it is rotated.[145]

Treatment is normally complete once the needle is withdrawn. In many cases, however, treatment may continue for weeks and months; this often turns out to be necessary particularly in the case of chronic ailments. According to doctors of the traditional school, the aim of acupuncture treatment does not consist merely in producing direct stimulation of the points of insertion, but also, and chiefly, in bringing about a harmonious functioning of the cortex.[146]

We will now briefly summarize the most popular insertion points and techniques. Chu Lien has noted the following:

1. Insertion of the needle into those points located symmetrically on, and common to, both left and right halves of the body.

2. Insertion of the needle at points with a similar effect on both the upper and lower extremities.

3. Simultaneous stimulation of the front of the body and the back. In this connection mention should be made of a combination of superficial and deep acupuncture, whereby points on the front part of the body and on the back, for example, are punctured at the same time, but to varying depths.

4. Simultaneous "internal" and "external" treatment, that is, stimulation of a *Yin* point and a *Yang* point at the same time.

5. A combination of direct and indirect stimulation, that is, simultaneous stimulation of a point near the seat of a disease and one remote from it.

6. Simultaneous stimulation of points along the spinal column and on the extremities.

7. In the case of varying symptoms, simultaneous stimulation at various points.

8. "General strengthening." This is based on simultaneous stimulation of the points treated for tonification purposes and those which "belong" to the illness in question.

9. Treatment in accordance with the "corresponding and changing times." This implies a change in the choice of points of tonification or sedation during the period of treatment.[147]

The decision as to which of the above methods of treatment is to be adopted depends on the patient's condition and the doctor's delicacy of touch. The above list therefore merely shows all of the possible methods and is not intended to indicate that all combinations must be used on any one patient.

113

TESTING TRADITION

Before we go on to a detailed account of the clinical results of acupuncture, it may be worthwhile briefly to summarize the present assessment of the traditions associated with it. Modern China sets great store on evaluating the methods of medical treatment which have been handed down and on continuing research into them.

The first of these aims is achieved through the publication of numerous works devoted to traditional medicine. The medical academies reprint the older books, together with commentaries, and thus make them available for modern research. The "Su Wên," "Ling Shu," the *Book of Ailments* (*Nan Ching*), and others have all been translated and published, together with commentaries, in recent years.

Quite a number of relevant research findings have also been published; and many modern publications, such as those by Chu Lien, Wang Hsüeh-tai, and others, in discussing ailments in modern terms, include the traditional terminology in brackets. In acupuncture theory, the traditional meridians are regarded as being of secondary importance, whereas greater attention is paid to the interconnection between the autonomic nervous system and the acupuncture points. As regards the various diseases, these are explained not according to the meridians, but according to the acupuncture points where treatment can best be applied. In such cases, modern technical anatomical terms are employed. Scientific publications pay little attention to the principle of *Yin* and *Yang,* or to the five elements, but nonetheless a thorough effort is being made to reappraise traditional medicine in the light of modern findings.

We should also consider too, before going on, why acupuncture and moxibustion are so popular throughout China (moxibustion will be taken up later in the book). The successes achieved by both of these methods of treatment are general knowledge in China, and nearly every Chinese citizen, as we have seen, is familiar with a few of the more effective acupuncture points. Furthermore, as the insertion of the needle does not particularly cause any pain, acupuncture treatment is willingly accepted by the people.

114

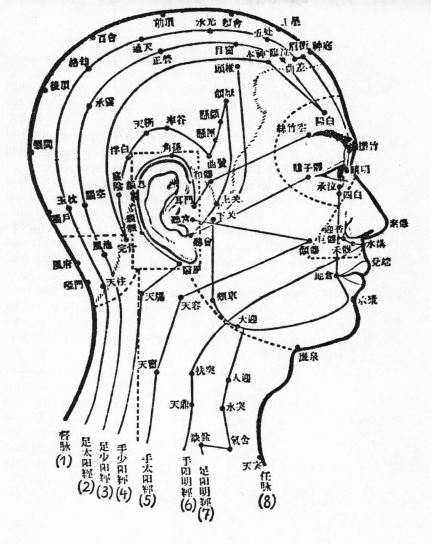

FIGURE 29
ACUPUNCTURE POINTS ON THE HEAD
(From a modern Chinese book on anatomy.)
The Chinese characters denote the various points, and the connecting lines between them represent the meridians. The dotted lines are merely for guidance.

We have numbered the individual meridians as follows: 1. *Tu-mai* meridian. 2. Bladder meridian. 3. Gall bladder meridian. 4. "Triple warmer" meridian. 5. Small intestine meridian. 6. Large intestine meridian. 7. Stomach meridian. 8 *Jên-mai* meridian.

115

In the first place, acupuncture is suitable for treating a wide variety of diseases, ranging from internal medicine to women's and children's ailments, from neurology to organotherapy. It is often used in combination with modern medical processes. It generally takes effect very quickly, particularly as regards the alleviation of pain, and often proves more efficacious than chemotherapeutical preparations. A further advantage is that the set of required instruments is rather simple. Acupuncture is not only easy to carry out, but very inexpensive as well. The methods of treatment can be learned comparatively easily, and can be carried out anywhere, since the only necessary preconditions are peace and quiet, and precautions against infection.[148]

The first general summary of the results achieved by acupuncture was made between 1951 and 1954 and covered the whole of China, including Inner Mongolia. Of 10,036 cases involving acupuncture, 8,063 were later evaluated. The statistical result was divided into four groups, namely, those which were cured, markedly improved, improved, and not improved. The total of all successfully treated cases averaged 92.47 per cent (see table).

Illnesses	Number of Cases	Cured	Markedly Improved and Improved	Not Improved	% Success
Nervous system	2236	652	1390	194	91.32
Locomotor system	2603	923	1532	148	94.31
Digestive system	1415	625	706	84	94.06
Blood circulation	375	54	248	73	80.53
Respiratory organs	504	166	306	32	93.65
Urogenital system	157	70	71	16	90.00
Gynecological cases	378	168	192	18	95.24
Sense organs	173	39	108	26	85.00
Skin diseases	44	21	22	1	97.73
Infectious diseases	142	90	43	9	93.66
Others	36	8	22	6	83.33
Total	8063	2816	4640	607	92.47

FIGURE 30
(From a modern Chinese book on anatomy.)
The Chinese characters denote the various points, and the connecting lines between them represent the meridians, which we have numbered as follows: 1. Spleen meridian. 2. Liver meridian. 3. Stomach meridian. 4. Kidney meridian. 5. Jên-mai meridian.

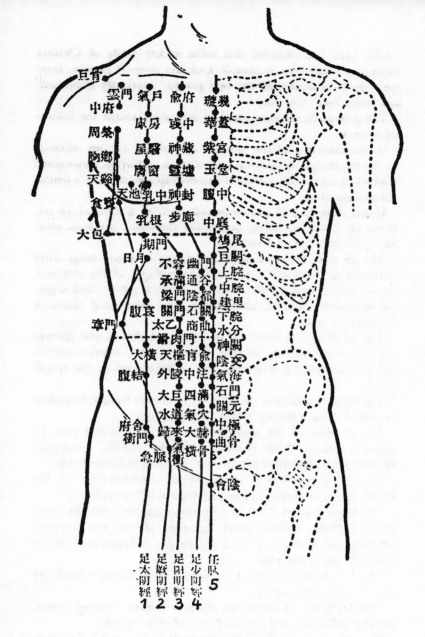

FIGURE 30
THE POINTS LOCATED ON THE FRONT OF THE TRUNK

117

Chu Lien has included this table in her study of Chinese medicine.[149] In order to provide a clearer over-all picture, however, we have combined the two groups "markedly improved" and "improved" into one.

The groups of illnesses listed in the table include the following ailments.

Under disorders of the *nervous system,* 42 various ailments are listed, including nervous convulsions, epilepsy, neurogenic headaches, meningitis, cerebral hemorrhage, Saint Vitus's dance, and poliomyelitis.

Under disorders of the *locomotor system,* a total of 16 ailments are listed, including periostitis, rheumatic diseases, muscular inflammation, and arthritis.

The 39 ailments listed under the *digestive system* range from toothache to esophagitis, and include prolapse of the stomach, excess gastric acid in the stomach, nervous gastric and digestive disorders, enteritis, cholecystitis, gallstones, and ulcers in the digestive tract.

The 18 disorders listed in the *blood circulation and haemapoietic systems* include anemia, heart diseases, arteriosclerosis, high blood-pressure, leukemia, and inflammation of the lymph glands.

The eight disorders of the *respiratory organs* include bronchial catarrh, asthma, pleurisy, sphagitis, and others.

The diseases of the *urogenital system* are divided into 17 ailments among them chronic nephritis, cystitis, spasmodic bladder pains, abnormal micturition, orchitis, and impotence.

The 14 *gynecological cases* include inflammation of the womb, irregular menstruation, and vaginal inflammation.

The large number (24) of ailments connected with the *sense organs* include, among others, keratitis, various eye diseases, inflammation of the outer and middle ear, inflammation of the nose (rhinitis), and others.

The commonest of the 11 types of *skin diseases* listed are eczema, boils, and rashes.

The ten types of *infectious diseases* include, among others, malaria, influenza, and various forms of tuberculosis.

The 13 types of *other ailments* include hormonal disorders, diabetes, and various kinds of toxicosis.

The *New Handbook of Acupuncture and Moxibustion* (*Hsin-pien Chên-chiu-hsüeh*), which appeared in Chungking in 1958, provides statistical data on 17,514 cases where acupuncture treatment was given. This shows that, even when this method, and no other, was used, good results were achieved in treating the following 26 ailments: malaria, inflammation of the intestines (*enteritis*), dysentery, bronchitis, insufficiency of the digestive system, trigeminal neuralgia, toothache, arthritis, tonsilitis, conjunctivitis, nervous stomach upsets, inflammation of the middle ear (*otitis media*), influenza, rheumatic diseases, sciatica, sacralgia, laryngitis, nettlerash (*urticaria*), kala-azar (*splenomegalia febrilis tropica*), muscular cramps, cholera, abnormal emission of seminal fluid (*spermatorrhea*), edema, epilepsy, radiculitis, and barley grain (*hordeolum* or style).

The highest number of cases involved malaria (5115 cases, percentage of success 90); nervous stomach upsets (2757 cases, percentage of success 63.9); rheumatic diseases (2467 cases, percentage of success 70.4); arthritis (1775 cases, percentage of success 55.6); trigeminal neuralgia (*nervus trigeminus, nervus facialis, and others*) (1041 cases, percentage success 97.4) and inflammation of the intestines (*enteritis*) (1,036 cases, percentage of success 88.3). The smallest number of cases concerned ejaculation of semen (*spermatorrhea*) (two cases, both of which were cured).[150]

It is still particularly difficult to explain how acupuncture and moxibustion take effect when treatment is being given for infectious diseases and disorders of the blood-forming organs (leukemia, anemia, and so on). In this connection we must await the results of further research.

Medical journals in China continually publish reports of new discoveries in the field of the traditional art of healing, all of which are supported by verifiable results. From these publications we learn, for example, that a success rate of 81 per cent was achieved in thirty districts in the treatment of malaria.[151] Between 1953 and 1955, some 98 cases of infantile paralysis were successfully treated by means of acupuncture in the Peking children's clinic. The success rate in cases of illness of less than a year's duration reached 100 per cent. Even in cases of one to two years' duration the success rate was still 92 per cent.

119

Cases of longer standing, on the other hand, resist acupuncture treatment.[152]

The Chinese medical journals also report on the treatment of appendicitis by means of acupuncture (success rate 92.3 per cent of 1202 cases) and the complete cure of 39 asthma cases.[153] There are numerous publications along similar lines, and Soviet Russian medical periodicals continue to report on new successes.[154]

In connection with acupuncture it is worth noting a particular curiosity which is well known in Hungary, where this present book was first published. In 1865 a small work entitled *Baunscheidtism* appeared on the Hungarian book market.[155] Its author, Karl Baunscheidt, was a machinist in Endenich, and the book was translated by P. M. Szabó. Baunscheidt recommended that both patients and doctors make use of an invention which he described as a "resuscitator." "This daring instrument," he wrote, "consists of a group of sharp-pointed needles which are inserted into the skin (a practically painless operation) in order to make artificial holes, thus creating a natural escape route for all the morbid matter which the malfunctioning of the skin has caused to accumulate at the painful spots and which is so injurious to the health."[156] The instrument is depicted in an illustration; it is similar to a special type of skin needle still used today in China. According to the invention, it was thanks to a mosquito that he hit upon the idea for his invention. The mosquito stung him in his rheumatic arm, which thereafter ceased to give him any pain. Baunscheidt carefully indicated the suitable points of insertion for various ailments. These included acupuncture points known to traditional Chinese medicine as well. The origin of the invention is made all the more doubtful by the author's categorical statement that the "Chinese needle-insertion method" is not identical with his own.

Having made this digression, we should also add that acupuncture therapy has been combined with modern medical methods of treatment as well, and that electric needles are also used (*electro-acupuncture, galvano-acupuncture*). Chu Lien has, in fact, become famous for her efforts to develop and extend the traditional acupuncture procedure.

120

5

MOXA TREATMENT (MOXIBUSTION)

WE have earlier noted that heat treatment or treatment by "burning" is associated with acupuncture both in modern literature and in what has come down to us by tradition, and that the two methods are often combined and applied at the same time. This explains why the clinical tests which we referred to in the previous chapter also included moxa treatment.

The process of healing by means of moxa treatment is also referred to by an older name, *moxibustion*. This word is compounded from the name for the Japanese plant *mogusa* (Latinized form: *moxa*), which is the same as *mugwort* (*artemisia vulgaris*), and the Latin root *uro* = to burn or scorch (see *comburere, combustus,* and *bustum* = a place where corpses are burned). As befits this nomenclature, the acupuncture points were formerly actually burned with "burning grass," that is to say, with a burning medical herb. Nowadays the points to be stimulated are merely warmed. The name *moxibustion* (*moxa burning*) is, it is true, still commonly used, but the term *moxa treatment* is more appropriate.

According to Professor Huard, the origin of this procedure probably pre-dates the insertion of stone needles, although the opposite view can be found in modern Chinese publications.[157] According to tradition, moxibustion was mainly developed in the northern part of China. Huard deduces from this that Stone Age man used moxa burning in order to ease the rheumatic pains caused by the cooler climate or the damp caves in which he lived.[158]

Certainly, the healing power of a warming fire was recognized

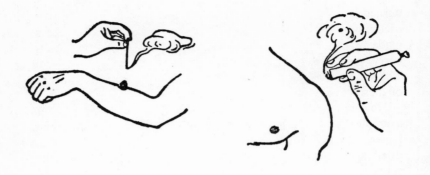

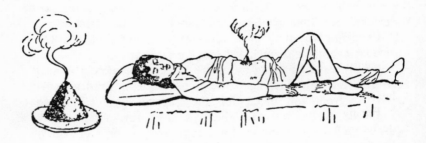

FIGURE 31
MOXA CONE, MOXA STICK, AND THEIR APPLICATION
Top left: moxa cone applied directly to the skin. *Top right:* heating by means of a moxa stick. *Bottom left:* moxa cone with base. *Bottom right:* application of a moxa cone with base.

even in very early times. Thus we find in the oldest collection of medical knowledge, *The Yellow Emperor's Classic of Internal Medicine,* references to moxibustion as a completely developed process.

In addition, any method of treatment involving warming presupposes knowledge of the stimulation points on the bodies of men and animals. Certain points are excluded from moxa treatment; they may be used only for acupuncture—and vice versa. Both old and new works list all these "forbidden" points.

In early times the points selected for treatment were also

burned by means of red-hot iron rods, a process which is today used only in veterinary surgery. In addition to iron rods, others made mainly from the rolled leaves of medicinal herbs (mulberry, ginger, aconite, mugwort, and so forth) were also used. The stimulation points were either burned or warmed by means of these glowing rod-formed leaves.

Nowadays various warming processes are in common use. For example, the medicinal herb is crushed and wrapped in special paper, lit, and held above the point which is to be warmed. The dried and rubbed herb can, however, also be made into the shape of a ball or cone and then placed on the actual point where treatment is to be applied. Once lit, the moxa cone remains on the skin until there is a danger of singeing or overheating, whereupon it is removed.

In certain cases the moxa cone or ball is also fitted with a special base; this will be discussed later.

In modern Chinese clinics it is mostly mugwort (*artemisia vulgaris*) leaves which are used, usually in the form of 10- to 12-centimeter-long sticks or else bean-sized cones and balls. The aim is to apply a pleasant warmth without causing a scorching heat.

For moxa treatment purposes the Japanese developed special devices consisting of small tubes, fitted with a handle, in which the powdered plant burned away. Similar devices are also to be found here and there in China.

The following details on the subject of moxa treatment are taken from modern Chinese publications:[159]

1. Three to five *moxa cones* or *balls* are required for one session; they may be lit and applied at the same time to various points on the body, or they may be lit and applied one after the other to the same point. Chronic conditions may require larger doses.

2. A *moxa stick* burns for four to five minutes. If a sedating effect is desired, the stick is held over the appropriate point on the body. This procedure can be used, for example, to remove a protective inhibition in the cerebral cortex. To achieve a tonifying effect the surface of the skin is lightly tapped with the glowing stick without overheating the point where the treatment is being applied. This is the so-called "bird-pecking" method.[160]

3. In the case of *moxa treatment with a ginger base,* a slab of fresh ginger is first placed on the point where treatment is to be applied, and the moxa cone is then set on top. When the ginger dries out it must be replaced. Generally speaking, this method is used for stomach ache, diarrhea with vomiting, and rheumatic pains in the limbs.

4. In the case of *moxa treatment with a garlic base,* a slab of fresh garlic is placed on the points where treatment is to be applied. A small hole is bored through the slab and the moxa cone is placed over it. Generally speaking, this method is employed to relieve pain and in certain cases for the treatment of pulmonary diseases (asthma, bronchitis, tuberculosis).

5. In the case of *moxa treatment with salt,* the point where treatment is to be applied is covered with salt and the moxa cone then placed on top. Whenever the salt becomes overheated, it is replaced. This method is normally used for abdominal pains, vomiting, and ailments caused by organic hypofunction. The aim is to compensate the "energy lack" in the afflicted organ.[161]

Moxa cones and sticks should be applied in varying dosages depending on the part of the body to be treated. For example, in the case of head punctures, the normal dosage is to allow the moxa to burn for 3–5 minutes, using sticks only, not cones. Other prescribed dosages are: on the chest, 3–5 minutes of steady heating with cones or 3–10 minutes with sticks; on the body, 5–20 minutes of steady heating with cones or 5–20 minutes with sticks; on the back, 3–10 minutes of steady heating with cones or 3–10 minutes with sticks.[162]

Correct positioning of the patient's body is of fundamental importance when moxa treatment is being given, in order that the points on the body are dealt with in the best possible way. Modern publications warn against scorching the patient's skin, and thus the old "scar" method is nowadays rejected, just as is burning by means of sulphur. Care must be taken to ensure that there are no sparks during treatment; the windows should also be opened to allow the dispersal of any smoke produced while the cone or stick is being burned. The fact that smoke is produced, incidentally, is the only disadvantage of this method of therapy.

After treatment has been carried out, all that is to be seen on the surface of the skin is, at most, a slight redness, and this soon vanishes. If any blisters appear, they are pierced with a sterile needle and rubbed with ointment.

The method of direct burning, which was formerly commonly used, left ugly scars on the skin, and these can still be seen today on elderly people in China and, more particularly, in Korea.

Modern medical science regards moxa treatment as a stimulation of the skin which is produced by heat and which may also, thanks to medical herbs (garlic, ginger, and others), possibly contain chemical properties. This opinion is shared by many doctors of the old school, including Wang Hsüeh-tai, who has both traditional and modern training. He does not, however, see any connection between moxa and *histamine treatment*.[163]

We already know that the vasodilative effect of skin stimulation reacts on the internal organs. This is explained by the close interconnection between these organs and special areas of the skin, whereby any disease of the former transmits a feeling of pain to the latter. Conversely, any stimulation of certain areas and points on the skin innervates the musculature and blood vessels and affects the relevant internal organs. These functional interrelationships also explain the efficacy of moxa treatment from a therapeutical point of view. The only slight difficulty consists in reconciling the traditional moxa points with the "skin areas" of modern medicine and incorporating them into one unified system.

6

RESPIRATORY THERAPY

RESPIRATORY therapy was already known in ancient China, and there is scarcely any other system of healing which is so closely interwoven with philosophical and religious movements.

An investigation of the origins of respiratory therapy is a difficult undertaking. This much may be immediately said, however, that the practices of magicians and hermits not only were intended to achieve heightened contemplation but had also a therapeutic purpose. This is confirmed by an inscription on twelve jade stones which has come down to us from the 6th century B.C.: "This is how breathing must be done: the breath is retained and collected. When it has collected, it expands. When it expands, it goes downwards. When it goes downwards, it becomes quiet. When it has become quiet, it grows firm. When it is firm, it begins to germinate. When it has germinated, it grows. When it has grown, it must be pressed back. When it has been pressed back, it reaches the crown of the head. At the top it presses against the crown of the head, down below it presses downwards. Whosoever follows this principle, lives; whosoever does the contrary, dies."[164]

It was only later that respiratory exercises were adopted by Taoism and Buddhism.[165] The terminology is mainly Taoist in origin, although partly Buddhist as well. We have discussed these two religious movements earlier in the book, and explained that Taoism, although it was a philosophy which had originated among the people themselves and was based on rational judgment, had nevertheless led in the course of time to what have occasionally been highly irrational interpretations and practices.

126

Even as early as the time of the first Emperor Ch'in Shih Huang-ti (3rd century B.C., Taoist magicians were living at the courts and seeking to find the "herb of eternal life" or elixir of immortality, the "Western paradise," and the philosopher's stone. Respiratory exercises were used in this connection in order to attain inner "immortality." Although medical works as well, including *The Yellow Emperor's Classic of Internal Medicine,* devote some attention to respiratory exercises,[166] it was Taoism which, by and large, first used this discipline as a type of therapy.

The spread of Buddhism in China also brought with it new aspects of respiratory exercises. It is a well-known fact that these formed an integral part of the *yoga* exercises of India, the cradle of Buddhism. Since Buddhism first reached China in the 1st century A.D., whereas the Chinese jade inscription on the subject of breathing dates back to the 6th century B.C., it may be assumed at the very least that there were no close connections between the formulation of the Indian and Chinese theories of respiration, and that both systems developed independently of another one. The Oriental scholar Henri Maspero is also of the opinion that the Taoist technique of breathing is not derived from Indian *yoga.*[167]

As Buddhism began to exert influence in China, the aim of the breathing exercises changed. Whereas the Taoists carried out these exercises, which had originally been aimed at producing a practical effect and were later used for religious purposes, in order to help them achieve material immortality and to "make the body light," the Buddhists' concern was of a spiritual kind: "purifying of the heart, calming of the spirit, so that each individual may be like Buddha."[168]

We also find the Taoist system in the work entitled *Diverse Notes on the Western Capital (Hsi Ching Tsa-chih)*, which dates from the 6th century A.D.[169] According to this book Liu An, the prince of Huainan, was greatly attached to his magicians, who could perform many kinds of tricks. One of them would draw a line on the ground, and out of the line water would begin to flow. Another would concentrate, then collect earth, and make a mountain out of it. Others through breathing could influence the weather and the seasons, summoning summer or winter as they wished. Others again could conjure rain or fog by sneezing or coughing. According to this report, Liu An himself finally vanished with the magicians and was never seen again.

Others who were concerned with respiratory therapy on a medical basis were Chang Chung-ching, who lived during the Han period, and Hua T'o, the discoverer of anaesthesia. The Taoist doctors devoted particular attention to their therapeutic and occult experiments. Their writings contain a mixture of both rational and irrational elements. For example, a work of the alchemist, magician, and physician Ko Hung (4th century A.D.), entitled *Pao P'u-tzû,* is a valuable treasury of precise observation of nature, but of Taoist superstition as well. The same can be said of the Taoist doctor and pharmacist T'ao Hung-ching (5/6th centuries A.D.), and the hermit doctor of the T'ang period, Sun Szû-miao. Li Shih-chên, the great 16th-century doctor and pharmacist, who was an enemy of superstition and combatted all mystical conceptions, likewise occupied himself with respiratory therapy.

GENERAL PRINCIPLES
OF RESPIRATORY THERAPY

The theory of respiratory therapy is based on the *Yin-Yang* principle, the doctrine of the five elements, and the traditional concept of the *Tsang* and *Fu* organs. Also of major importance is the age-old *"Ch'i"* theory (*Ch'i = breath, air, energy*), which we have already described. Here *Ch'i* still has its original meaning of *"air."* Later, the term also came to include inhalation and exhalation, together with the relevant human emotions, and it has nowadays acquired a particularly neurophysiological meaning, in the sense of affecting nervous activity. Thus a person can, for example, have *Ch'i* for walking and for sensations of warmth and cold.[170]

The aim of respiratory therapy exercises is to produce *Ch'i* (*Ch'i-kung = preparation of Ch'i*). Consequently, the respiratory exercises do not consist only of simple inhalation and exhalation; they require the participation of the entire automatic nervous system and consciousness. Each exercise includes "inner activity" (*Nei-kung*) and "outer strengthening" (*Ch'iang-*

128

chuang-kung). The two exercise components together are referred to as the "way to the preservation of life" (*Yang-shêng*).[171]

The term *"T'u-na"* is also commonly found in older writings; this is an abbreviation of the Taoist expression *"T'u-ku Na-hsin,"* "breathe the old out and the new in." The term *"Tao-yin"* (to lead, leadership) is also Taoist in origin, and signifies combined respiratory and gymnastic exercises.

According to ancient theory, the body "preserves" the *Ch'i,* which also circulates in the five elements. These in turn are similarly present in "heaven and earth." The body, however, is at the same time the "keeper of the five elements" and, consequently, of the "energy" active in these elements as well.

Ch'i influences the interplay between *Yin* and *Yang* and the relationships between the "five elements" not only in all of the cosmos, but in each individual. *Ch'i* incites the inner organs to activity, and it follows, therefore, that every illness (that is, disturbance of the organic harmony) can be attributed to inadequate circulation or lack of *Ch'i.*[172]

The aim of both respiratory and gymnastic exercises is therefore to stimulate the harmonizing "circulation" by means of inner "passive" and outer "active" effect.

According to tradition, an exercise of the "outer parts" alone without demanding anything of the "inner parts" is not sufficient. Exercise of the "outer parts" means moving the arms, legs, trunk, and head. The aim of the "inner" exercises, on the other hand, is to influence the internal organs knowns as *Fu* and *Tsang* and thereby to affect the entire nervous system. Activation of the musculature is comparatively simple, since the limbs can be moved arbitrarily, but generally speaking it is not normally possible to influence the internal organs by will power alone. Here we come back to the importance of the respiratory exercises, because with their help it is possible to influence the control of the organs. The two phases of the breathing process move the diaphragm, and its displacement enables the internal organs to be affected. If the respiratory exercises are correctly carried out, then "the internal organs gradually obey the dictates of the will and their functioning can be controlled."[173]

Modern interpretation of the traditional art of healing suggests that the special features of respiratory therapy are as follows.

1. Basically, the patient heals himself. The doctor who controls the exercises merely helps him to overcome his illness. The success obtained by means of the exercises increases the patient's optimism—a very important consideration, particularly in cases of ailments which are associated with depression.

2. Respiratory therapy is concerned with "internal" exercises, in contrast to "external" gymnastic ones. Since the patient will not normally be used to "internal" exercises, the first thing to do is to establish a connection between breathing and this special form of consciousness. This requires patience and confidence in the therapist on the part of the patient, who must likewise display equability of temperament and not expect dramatic results. As the result of regular respiratory exercises, synesthetic sensations may occur after a certain period of time, such as *chromopsy* (color vision) or a feeling of weightlessness,— transcendental states to which certain Taoists and Buddhists have attached great importance.

3. Due account must be taken of the patient's mentality, normal diet, and environment. It can therefore be useful to combine respiratory therapy with other methods of treatment. Any pseudo-religious ecstasies on the part of the patient or— and these often occur in conjunction with this type of therapy— occult hallucinations must either be avoided or corrected.

4. The effect of the respiratory exercises on the functions of the internal organs is a slow one, and it is therefore important for the exercises to be carried out in a natural and unconstrained manner. Any conscious striving after quick success, or restless, impatient exercising, can do untold harm. Not only is the desired success jeopardized; harmful physiological changes may also be caused. It is thus important that the patient follow his doctor's instructions and not merely carry out the exercises as he himself thinks fit.

5. Respiratory therapy includes both "movement and rest," both components being essential for the achievement of a state of equilibrium.

Day-long relaxation is as bad for the health as incessant exercise.

6. A very important factor is the provision of an equable, quiet environment. It is essential that there should be a peaceful atmosphere in the sanatorium so that the patient will be able to relax. The therapist must also closely watch the patient's appetite in order to ensure that the success of the exercises is not jeopardized either by hunger or surfeit.

7. If the patient feels tired during the exercises, he should desist, for overexertion can have unpleasant consequences. If, on the other hand, a pleasant feeling of relaxation develops during the exercises, this means that the desired state of "repose" has set in. Chinese doctors have described this state in terms of modern physiology as one in which the cerebral cortex has achieved the condition of *special protective inhibition*.

8. It is possible that dyskinetic phenomena may occur during the exercises as a result of "inner energy." This refers to natural reactions which, together with special faculties of perception, are regarded as typical of a certain degree of inhibition of the cortex. That is to say, if a comparatively serious degree of inhibition already extends over a large part of the cortex, and the center of movement suddenly receives a stimulus, then this impulse is reflected in disconnected movements on the part of the patient. The therapeutic view is that it is extremely harmful to induce such movements deliberately.

These movement phenomena are of secondary importance. The patient should therefore strive to maintain his state of repose; he must not admit that the desired psychosomatic state of equilibrium is affected by such movement mechanisms.[174]

METHODS OF RESPIRATORY THERAPY

The technique of respiratory therapy cannot be learned from books; the doctor administering the treatment must therefore himself be well experienced in breathing exercises in order to be in a position to brief the patient and advise him correctly in cases of difficulty. This is why institutes where respiratory therapy is given employ only doctors who thoroughly understand the exercises, who know how to brief the patients, and who are also trained in modern medical knowledge.

131

The exercises are carried out in accordance with three important principles.

First of all, there must be *relaxation* and *repose* (*Sung-ching Wei Chu*). Relaxation here means a relaxing of the entire body, whereas repose implies tranquillity of the spirit. Both external and internal peace and quiet are consequently absolutely essential prior to the exercises. According to traditional medicine, the patient's spirit is quietened more easily if his muscles are relaxed; conversely, if the spirit remains tense during the exercises, this tension is transmitted to the musculature.

The second important principle is the *association of respiration with attention* (*I-ch'i Ho-i*). Breathing should be easy and gentle, whereas the attention should be riveted on one object only. According to Chinese doctors, there are many people who regard respiratory exercises as a kind of "work." Thus some thrust out the abdomen and purposely suppress the intake of air —so that the patient can neither breathe properly nor control his respiration. Traditional teaching requires the very opposite; the attention should be controlled by breathing, and not the other way around.

The third important principle is the *interaction of exercising and resting* (literally, "feeding") (*Lien-yang Hsiang-chien*). The traditional doctors are of the opinion that patients, generally speaking, know more about exercising than they do about resting. Thus they must learn to relax, and thus be enabled not only to carry out the exercises but to interrupt or leave off with them altogether in accordance with the requirements of the organism. The person doing the exercises may be sure that Nature, in her capacity as the careful controller of all vital processes, will endorse any psychosomatic harmonization. The interplay of exercise and rest is thus of extreme importance as far as respiratory therapy is concerned. What usually happens is that those who think they know everything and can do everything go ahead and practice the exercises unrestrainedly. "The effect is as if we were to pile fresh logs on a well-burning fire—which is already sending out a good heat—so as to make it burn more fiercely." The patient should therefore never exert himself; every imbalance is to be avoided.[175]

The breathing exercises are carried out in various postures.

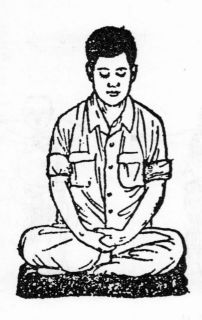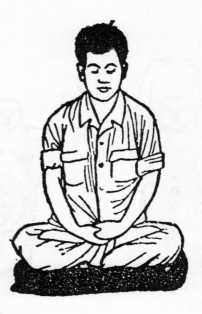

FIGURE 32
SITTING POSTURES FOR BREATHING EXERCISES
Left: instep of one foot resting on the opposite thigh.
Right: both insteps resting on the thighs.

Common ones are lying on one's side, lying on one's back (with a cushion under the head), sitting upright, and standing. The sitting postures are the "Turkish position," which is very common in the East, and variations of it. The base on which the patient is lying or sitting should be firm yet comfortable.

Once the correct posture is adopted, the exercise begins under the therapist's direction. The introductory exercise is always one from the "inner strengthening" series; the patient first of all calms his body by untensing his muscles one after the other or, more precisely expressed, he lets himself relax. This release of tension takes place in a set sequence, beginning at the head and ending at the toes. The doctors of the old school emphasize the necessity of untensing not only the muscles and joints but also the internal organs and the nervous system as well.

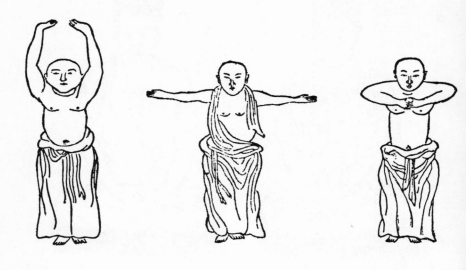

FIGURE 33
"OUTER" EXERCISES COMBINED WITH BREATHING EXERCISES
Representation of an "outer" exercise combined with a series of breathing
exercises, extracted from the *Book of Light Muscles* (Ch'ing period).

It is only then that the breathing exercises proper begin. The
patient first of all breathes in his own natural way, and then does
so more and more deeply in stages until he is practicing diaphragmatic respiration, but still gently and easily. All this time
he is breathing deeply through his nose and centering his attention on the umbilical region. To facilitate the procedure the patient should think of a definite word (as of "quiet") while he is
breathing in and out. The attention can also be concentrated on
other parts of the body, for example, the tips of the toes.

The *"combined forms of internal conserving exercises"* consist, for example, in breathing out through the open mouth and
directing attention to the head. This relaxes the head and neck
musculature. After exhalation through the mouth comes inhalation through the nose. Then the previously described exercise
is repeated, but with the difference that attention is now con-

centrated on the shoulders and arms, the muscles of which are consciously relaxed by the exhalation. The exercise continues in this fashion until the toe musculature is untensed.

There are several variations of the "internal conserving exercises." For example, the patient may adopt a composed posture, contemplate the end of his nose as he breathes in and out, relax completely, and think of the same word each time he draws breath. This exercise is termed "harmony and peace." Another variation is to allow the attention to "dwell" on the umbilical region or on the legs and to inhale through the nose and exhale through the mouth.

The important interaction between exercising and resting occurs as follows: midway through the exercise the patient ceases all deliberate activity for a short time, allows his attention to center exclusively on the umbilical region, and remains so for several minutes. The traditional doctors describe this as "composure."

Another possible method of resting consists of letting oneself go completely, allowing the mind to relax without thinking, and remaining in this half trance-like state which is neither "dream nor wakefulness." If this period of rest continues, it can easily develop into sleep.[176]

EFFECT OF THE EXERCISES

At this point we should inquire into the practical significance of such exercises, for at first sight they may seem to be a mere blend of medicine with the traditional Far Eastern technique of withdrawing from the world and "contemplating one's navel."

The Buddhist term for "sitting still" (*Ch'ing-tso*), or the Taoist word for "composure" (*Shou*) or for "resting" (*Yang*), no longer have today an exclusively religious significance. The simple method of "sitting still" or "resting" is, it is true, still practiced by members of these two religions, and it also plays a role in some areas of Christianity (as in the meditation exercises of the Trappists), and in other religions as well; but this fact does not thereby exclude any medical value from the exercises. The Chinese realized this fact, and gradually began to separate the medically usable nucleus of the exercises from their religious connotations. Today the breathing exercises can be summarized as follows.[177]

In most cases the patient's cerebral cortex is in a heightened state of excitement. After the appropriately selected exercises have been carried out, however, his general condition is good; his external and internal tensions have diminished and he has become more balanced and serene.

1. *Relaxation* remains the basis of every breathing exercise. Its value can be appreciated only by those who have actually carried out the exercises over a period of time.

The breathing exercises are normally done prior to eating or sleeping or if the patient is in pain. Experience has also proved that they can control irregularities in blood pressure.

2. *"The internal conserving exercises"* help to set the mind at ease. They also make "rough" breathing quieter, gentler, and more even, and heavy breathing light and easy. The "conserving" exercises also facilitate activity of the intestines and improve the appetite. In addition, they can stimulate and regulate the circulation of the blood.

The cerebral cortex relaxes more easily in a state of inhibition induced in such a way. It has also been observed that diaphragmatic breathing has a beneficial effect on the functioning of the diaphragm itself; this is quite important as regards treatment of prolapse of the stomach, since the stomach itself is pressed upwards by an increase in abdominal pressure.

3. It is also known that tensions occurring in exercise are released thanks to the *interplay* of "exercise and rest." Such interplay is of special importance to physically weakened people, for whom too much exercise is not suitable, so that they may overcome their exhausted condition.

"EXTERNAL" STRENGTHENING EXERCISES

According to doctors of the traditional school, "external" exercises encourage good posture and also help to prevent or combat illness.

We have already described the most suitable postures for en-

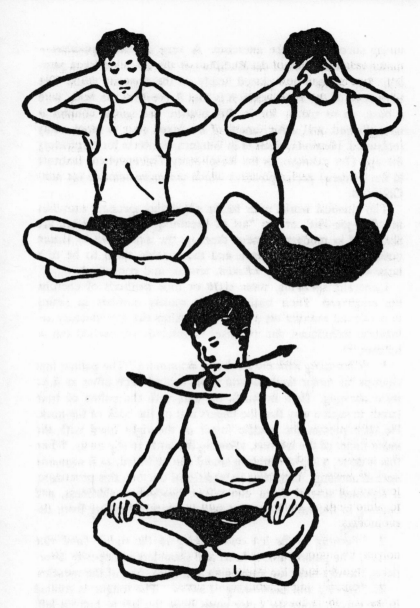

FIGURE 34
THREE "EXTERNAL" EXERCISES
Above: "champing with the teeth and drumming."
Below: "turning to the right, looking to the left."

137

suring success with the exercises. A very common position—shown often in idols of the Buddha—is the so-called lotus position: feet crossed and placed firmly on the opposite thigh. The advantage of the lotus position is that it provides the body with a base, so to speak, for in this posture the spinal column is strengthened, and achievement of a relaxed state is more easily facilitated. However, doctors in Western sanatoria for respiratory therapy (for example, in the Respiratory Therapeutical Institute in the Crimea) prefer postures which are more suitable for non-Orientals.

The classical works refer to the physiotherapeutical exercises as *"Tao-yin-shu"* or the "art of breathing." The exercises are also used in modern Chinese therapy, the aim being to loosen both joints and musculature and thus enable them to be to a large extent consciously relaxed, tensed, and controlled.

Generally speaking, some eight or nine methods of exercise are employed. Their basic posture mostly consists in sitting in a relaxed manner on a firm base. After the introductory relaxation techniques, the exercises themselves are carried out as follows.[178]

1. *"Champing with the teeth and drumming."* The patient first champs his molar teeth several times against each other as if he were chewing. Then he holds his ears with the palms of both hands in such a way that the fingers rest on the back of the neck. He then presses the middle finger of the right hand with the index finger of the left one, allowing the latter to slip away. When this is done, a slight vibrating sound can be heard, as if someone were drumming. According to traditional doctors, this procedure, if repeated several times, can relieve headaches, giddiness, and buzzing in the ears; it is even said to prevent hearing from deteriorating.

2. *"Turning to the left and looking to the right"* (and vice versa). The patient moves head and shoulders in opposite directions, thereby inducing slackening and relaxation of the muscles.

3. *"Stirring and swallowing of saliva."* The tongue is rotated in the mouth along the outer gums from top left to bottom left, after which it is rubbed against the palate. The abundance of saliva produced removes any bitter taste in the mouth and also helps digestion.

138

4. *"Massage of the sacral region with both hands."* The patient first warms the palms of his hands by rubbing them and then massages both sides of the sacral region with a downwards motion of the outstretched arms. This exercise can be used to relieve sacralgia and menstrual pains.

5. *"Stretching out the arms."* The patient clenches his fists, stretches his arms out at his sides, and then moves them towards the trunk as if he were pulling something towards himself. This exercise helps to straighten the spinal column.

6. *"Double winds."* Both hands are clenched and placed on the chest, and the shoulders and arms are then rotated backwards. This exercise stimulates the respiratory organs.

7. *"Raising the palms."* The patient stretches his arms forwards with the palms upwards. He then bends his forearms till the palms of his hands are directly in front of his face. This exercise encourages smooth functioning of the stomach and bowels.

8. *"Relaxed muscles and loose joints."* The patient remains seated, stretches out his legs, lowers his head "in a devout manner," stretches out his arms, and touches his toes. This exercise is prescribed for relaxation and for stimulation of the circulation.

All of these exercises should be carried out slowly, quietly, and physiologically, and above all without any undue exertion. Together with others which we shall describe later, they are used regularly by many of the Chinese people both to prevent illness and to achieve a general well-balanced state of health.

The traditional art of healing has developed interesting rules for the patient's daily routine, and, although critical investigation has shown much of what has survived to be pure speculation, many of the age-old precepts have a nucleus of sound commonsense which is still valid today. An example is provided in the instructions laid down for the treatment of liver and spleen sufferers in a book entitled *A Thousand Ducat Prescriptions* (*Ch'ien Chin Fang*), compiled by the Taoist doctor Sun Szû-miao (5th/6th centuries A.D.). We shall compare them with the daily routine of a modern Chinese sanatorium for respiratory therapy.

Sun Szû-miao[179] states the following: "A patient suffering from a liver complaint will practice *K'o respiration*. Patients with this nature of illness are depressed, sad, prone to worry; their head and eyes are painful; the face is livid in color, greenish-bluish. If these sufferers dream that they see a man dressed in greenish clothing, or of a lion, tiger, or leopard that has come to terrify people, then *K'o* respiration must be applied as a cure—the large *K'o* and the small *K'o* 30 times each. In addition, the 'left and right bodily exercise' (*Tao-yin*) must also be carried out 360 times. This will produce a cure."

Sufferers from ailments of the spleen are recommended to use the *"Hsi"* method of respiration, as follows: "Take 81 deep breaths at midnight, 72 at cock-crow, 62 at dawn, 54 at sunrise, 45 during *Ch-ên* (in the morning between 7 and 9 o'clock), and 36 during *Szû* (in the forenoon between 9 and 11 o'clock). Whosoever follows this advice should also carry out the 'left and right bodily exercise' prior to the deep breathing procedure, 360 times . . ."[180]

Figures played an important part in alchemy and cabbalistic lore. Odd figures were *Yang,* even ones *Yin;* hence the number of breaths had to be odd or even depending on the time of day. We now know that such notions have no real foundation. Nor does one necessarily have to suffer from a liver complaint to dream of wild beasts and dangerous people. Nevertheless, the division of the respiratory exercises according to the time of day, together with the descriptions of the symptoms which accompany diseases of the liver, provide a summary of what was then understood about the possible causes of illness.

What happens when a patient enters a modern Chinese sanatorium? First of all, his heart, lungs, stomach, blood pressure, and other functions are thoroughly examined. The patient is then informed of his condition, and a recuperative schedule is established. An introductory period of exercises determines whether or not respiratory therapy would be beneficial to him at all.

During his stay in the sanatorium the patient is subjected to a daily routine which ensures maintenance of the necessary peace and quiet. The patient keeps a diary in writing, including a description of each phase of his illness, together with notes on any progress or signs of relapse.

140

After the anamnesis is complete, the patient is shown how to relax. (Modern Chinese doctors are generally of the opinion, of course, that relaxation alone cannot produce a cure.) He is required to carry out the relaxation exercises five times daily during his entire stay in the sanatorium, 20 to 30 minutes each time.

Generally speaking, a start can be made on the "internal exercises" within five days; each exercise lasts 30 to 50 minutes. As the cure proceeds, "combined exercises" are added. The patient always carries out his exercise in a room full of fresh air but without draughts and at the correct temperature. All conversation ceases some 20 minutes before the exercise begins, in order to induce the necessary concentration.

The daily routine is as follows:

6:00– 6:20 A.M.	rise, wash, make bed
6:20– 7:00	sport, massage or exercises carried out slowly
7:00– 8:00	breakfast, clean out rooms
8:00– 8:50	first series of exercises
9:00–10:30	physical work (as in gardening), consumption of fruit or glucose
10:40–11:25	second series of exercises
11:45–12:10 P.M.	lunch
12:30– 2:20	rest in bed
2:30– 3:20	third series of exercises
3:20– 3:30	consumption of fruit or glucose
3:30– 4:20	gardening or other open-air work
4:30– 5:20	fourth series of exercises
5:40– 6:00	supper
6:00– 8:00	own choice of activity
8:00– 8:50	fifth series of exercises
9:00	bed.[181]

The patient is subjected to repeated examination until he leaves the sanatorium. In particular, he must commit his experience to paper, and his notes are included with the medical findings and clinical history.[182]

Various troubles may arise in the course of the exercises due to incorrect posture, respiratory errors, insufficient concentration, or synesthetic sensations. Thorough methods of overcoming these troubles have been developed, however, and they

141

have proved their worth in actual practice; they normally consist of a combination of modern procedures, notably medicamental treatments, and the traditional methods (acupuncture, moxibustion, massage, and so on).[183]

ANALYSIS OF THE RESULTS OF TREATMENT

So far we have discussed only the practical application of respiratory therapy and merely touched here and there on basic questions of principle. In Western countries, Chinese respiratory therapy has not yet been put into practice; in fact, apart from its historical form (Stiefvater), it has hardly been described at all. The only Chinese-style sanatorium in Europe, for example, is in the Soviet Union.[184]

The way in which respiratory therapy works is explained away by modern Chinese scientists on the basis of Pavlov's theory of the nervous system. They have concluded that the concepts of illness which emerged in olden times were superstitious in form only, and that they were basically, by and large, correct and compatible with Pavlov's theory.[185]

In the opinion of Chinese scientists the respiratory and relaxation exercises represent methods of transforming the patient's cerebral cortex into a state of high-degree harmony (protective inhibition). The patient's organic activity is under *higher* control when the cerebral cortex is functionally equable. The organism's powers of resistance to pathogenic agents are thereby strengthened and the general state of health regains its "equilibrium." The respiratory exercises strengthen the patient's defense mechanism and the physical exercises also stimulate the internal organs.

According to Pavlov, the cerebral cortex not only controls the equilibrium of the organs; it also affects their regeneration. This is why various functional disorders of the internal organs can be favorably influenced by means of respiratory exercises.

Those members of the physiological team of the First Medical Academy in Shanghai who have been carrying out research into respiratory therapy have proved by experiment that the successes achieved by the Chinese in this field can be accounted for scien-

142

tifically. They have further proved that exhalation and inhalation have varying effects on the organism. Exhalation stimulates the parasympathetic part of the nervous system, whereas inhalation does the same for the sympathetic part. This would also confirm what has happened in actual practice, namely, that ailments due to disorders of the autonomic nervous system can be cured by respiratory exercises.[186]

In present-day China, doctors who have received modern training but respect the old traditions consider it essential, in the interests of research, to develop precise instruments which will enable the functional mechanism of respiratory therapy to be measured. Current investigations are greatly helped by the *electroencephalograph* and the *acupuncture point ammeter,* the latter of which is much used in acupuncture research. According to Chinese doctors, the main task today is to make a more precise examination of the connection between conscious breathing and unconscious organic activity, together with the effect which this relationship may have on the healing process.

In modern China there are numerous medical establishments where respiratory therapy is practiced, notably those in Tangshan and Shanghai, which have a specially fine reputation. A similar establishment was set up in the Soviet Union, in the Crimea. The results achieved with 500 patients who underwent traditional Chinese respiratory therapeutical treatment were published in 1958.[187] The Shanghai sanatorium was founded in 1957, mainly for the treatment of patients suffering from stomach and intestinal ailments, whereas the one in Tangshan chiefly treats consumptives.

The following table shows the 1958 statistics for the Shanghai sanatorium.[188]

Illness	Number of Cases Treated	Completely Cured	Markedly Improved	Improved	Not Improved	% of Positively Influenced Cases
Duodenal ulcers	21	13	7	1	0	100
Duodenal ulcers with prolapse of the stomach	12	4	6	2	0	100
Prolapse of the stomach	8	5	2	1	0	100
Total	41	22	15	4	0	100

The same sanatorium also investigated the effects of respiratory therapy on special symptoms associated with stomach and intestinal ailments.[189]

Symptom	Number of Cases Treated	Completely Cured	Improved	Not Improved	% of Positively Influenced Cases
Lack of appetite	15	13	2	0	100
Depression	4	4	0	0	100
Nervous exhaustion ("nervous breakdown")	8	8	0	0	100
Eructation	32	19	13	0	100
Vomiting of gastric acid	27	20	6	1	96
Stomach pains	40	22	16	2	95
Distension of the abdomen	39	26	12	1	97
Malignant vomiting (hyperemesis)	2	1	0	1	50
Black stool	3	3	0	0	100

Upon leaving the sanatorium, the patients are X-rayed. The results achieved by the Shanghai sanatorium in 1958 were as follows.[190]

Illness	Number of Cases Treated	Completely Cured	Improved	Not Improved	% of Positively Influenced Cases
Duodenal ulcers	15	2	8	5	66.6
With prolapse of the stomach	3	1	2	0	100.0
Prolapse of the stomach	6	2	3	1	83.3
Total	24	5	13	6	75.0

It should be noted, however, with regard to these statistics, that it was impossible in many cases to make an exact assessment, since many patients were not in possession of X-ray records when admitted, although they had suffered from their complaints for years.

144

In order to give a complete picture let us quote from some case histories.

1. Chu, X. Y., workman, 28, record #57. Illness began prior to 1954. Complaints: pains in the abdominal region, painful vomiting. It was possible to alleviate pains by medical treatment, but they became worse in June 1956; according to the findings of the Sixth Municipal Hospital in Shanghai the stool contained blood, and the presence of a duodenal ulcer was confirmed. After five months of hospital treatment the patient was discharged as cured. A year later the stool again contained blood. The patient was told to stay at home for six months and rest. In the four months prior to admission to the sanatorium he experienced continual pain in the stomach and lumbar region, continued to bring up gastric acid, and was subject to fits of giddiness. On March 13, 1958, he was referred to the Sanatorium for Respiratory Therapy. On admission, his face had a yellowish tinge, his weight was 56.5 kg., the number of red blood corpuscles was 4,140,000 and the percentage of hemoglobin was 83. X-ray examination revealed a duodenal ulcer, and the abdominal region was painful and sensitive to pressure. Diagnosis: duodenal ulcer (*ulcus duodeni*).

After the general relaxation exercises the headaches diminished. On March 23 the "combined" exercises began, the patient's appetite increased, his physical condition improved, and the lumbar pains decreased. Once he had fully mastered the technique of diaphragmatic breathing the abdominal pains ceased. On April 5 he began "internal" strengthening exercises (eight light breaths per minute). The symptoms of disease vanished completely. The patient's complexion was rosy, his weight had risen to 62.5 kg., the number of red blood corpuscles was 4,510,000 and the percentage of hemoglobin was 90. The X-ray examination revealed that the duodenal ulcer was completely cured. The stomach was no longer sensitive to pressure, and on August 17, 1958, after four months' treatment, Chu was able to leave the sanatorium, cured.

2. Wei, X. Y., 35, male nurse, record #58. Complaint: pains in the abdominal region after meals. Patient had been complaining of irregular digestion for 18 years. Since 1955 the abdominal and intestinal pains had been increasing. His condition im-

proved after he had been given medicine. In March 1957, the Central Hospital in the Huangfu Region diagnosed from an X-ray examination that the patient had a duodenal ulcer and prolapse of the stomach. From March 1958 onwards, he complained of continual abdominal pains and distension, excessive gastric acid, and bloody stool. He went to the First General Hospital in Shanghai, where he received treatment with traditional Chinese medicaments as an out-patient; as a result, the pains subsided. On March 27, 1958, he was referred to the Shanghai Sanatorium for Respiratory Therapy. On admission the abdominal region was sensitive to pressure, his weight was 51 kg., and the lower part of the stomach had sunk nine centimeters below the line of the pelvis. Number of red blood corpuscles: 4,300,000; percentage of hemoglobin: 85. Diagnosis: prolapse of the stomach.

After the first relaxation exercises the excess of gastric acid was reduced and the patient's complaints about pains in the abdominal region became fewer. On April 2 the "combined exercises" began, and this brought about a further improvement in his condition. On April 14 the "internal" strengthening exercises commenced, whereupon the pains ceased completely, the stomach gave no further cause for complaint, appetite was good, and weight increased. An examination on July 4 revealed that the number of red blood corpuscles was 4,340,000 and the percentage of haemoglobin 86. On July 16 the patient's weight was 53.5 kg. An X-ray examination showed that the lower part of the stomach was now only three centimeters below the line of the pelvis. On July 20 the patient left the sanatorium, cured.[191]

The Tangshan sanatorium, directed by Liu Kui-chên, treats consumptives mainly, but also takes patients with neurovegetative disorders and diseases of the gastro-intestinal tract. In 1957, Doctor Kui-chên published *The Practice of Respiratory Therapy* (*Ch'i-kung Liao-fa Shih-chien*), according to which some 500 patients were successfully treated in eight years using respiratory therapy alone. Unfortunately, no statistics are given.

The Shanghai Sanatorium for Respiratory Therapy also makes use of scientific techniques. Its staff is particularly in-

146

terested, for example, in the changes in electrical potential of the acupuncture points on the body with reference to respiratory therapy.

The main aim of the research group in the Sanatorium for Respiratory Therapy is to solve the question whether or not the harmonization achieved by means of respiratory therapy can be proved by experiment. An electroencephalograph and an "acupuncture point micro-ammeter" are now being used for investigation purposes. A combined machine is currently being developed from these two devices.

As an illustration, we quote below data calculated from 123 cases of consumption and 49 cases of stomach trouble. The index figures were measured at the *Yüan* points on the main meridians by means of the "acupuncture point micro-ammeter." The *Yüan* points, it is well known, represent a bridge between the tonification and sedation points on the various meridians.

MEASURED VALUES FOR CONSUMPTIVES.[192]

Measuring Point	Meridian	Index Figure
T'ai-yüan	lung	47/48
Ho-ku	large intestine	42/43
Shên-mên	heart	37/37
Wan-ku	small intestine	44/46
T'ai-pai	spleen	43/45
T'ai-ch'i	kidney	41/41
T'ai-ch'ung	liver	45/46
Ching-ku	bladder	40/40
Ch'iu-hsü	gall bladder	30/31
Ch'ung-yang	stomach	45/45

According to this table, the relatively highest index figures (47/48) are to be found on the lung meridian, and the lowest (30/31) on the gall bladder meridian.

According to the next table, the index figures (55/56) for the spleen meridian are relatively high, and the figure for the stomach meridian is also larger than the corresponding entry in the previous table.

It is interesting to note the differences in measured values

147

Measuring Point	Meridian	Index Figure
T'ai-yüan	lung	50/52
Ho-ko	large intestine	45/46
Shên-mên	heart	37/38
Wan-ku	small intestine	48/49
T'ai-pai	spleen	55/56
T'ai-ch'i	kidney	45/46
T'ai-ch'ung	liver	49/50
Ching-ku	bladder	44/46
Ch'iu-hsü	gall bladder	32/36
Ch'ung-yang	stomach	51/52

after respiratory exercises have been carried out. Thus after a 40-minute period of exercise, index figures show that the previous wide scatter has been reduced and that the results now tend to form a well-balanced, average pattern. At the same time there are increased figures, particularly in respect of the lung, large intestine, gall bladder, and bladder meridians, all of which points towards a harmonizing tendency.

COMPARATIVE VALUES BEFORE AND AFTER
THE GENERAL RESPIRATORY EXERCISES.[194]

Measuring Points	Meridian	Index Figure Before Exercises	Index Figure After Exercises
T'ai-yüan	lung	7/7	20/35
Ho-ku	large intestine	7/7	42/50
Shên mên	heart	8/12	25/30
Wan-ku	small intestine	21/21	35/35
Ta-ling	"controller of the heart"	8/14	20/30
Yang-chê	"triple warmer"	5/5	10/42
T'ai-pai	spleen	25/50	52/55
T'ai-ch'i	kidneys	19/20	36/42
T'ai-ch'ung	liver	15/16	44/46
Ching-ku	bladder	46/63	50/63
Ch'iu-hsü	gall bladder	5/6	14/14
Ch'ung-yang	stomach	11/15	21/21

The following table shows that the "conserving" relaxation exercises can also produce beneficial results.

Measuring Point	Index Figure Before Exercise	Index Figure After Exercise
Yin-chiao	53	40
Ch'i-hai	50	40
Shih-mên	56	40
Kuan-yüan	57	40
Chung-chi	50	40
Ch'ü-ku	50	40

The next table shows the results of an interesting experiment: the "mental" pronunciation of various single-syllabic words during exhalation produces different index figures.[196]

Experiments	*T'ai-yüan* (lung)	*Shên-mên* (heart)	*Yang-che* (triple warmer)	*T'ai-ch'i* (kidney)	*T'ai-pai* (spleen)	*T'ai-ch'ung* (liver)
1st experiment: mental	74/74	35/38	58/60	48/48	55/57	57/60
Values prior to the experiment· repetition of "*Hsi*" twelve times	74/78	40/54	64/68	56/56	58/62	54/60
2nd experiment: mental repetition of "*Ch'ui*" twelve times	50/50	35/36	44/48	43/44	42/45	42/44
3rd experiment: five minutes' rest	50/51	36/39	44/48	40/45	42/46	42/45
4th experiment: mental repetition of "*K'o*" twelve times	52/54	24/26	46/47	42/42	42/43	46/46
5th experiment: five minutes' rest	48/49	36/37	42/44	38/38	39/40	36/36

This table seems to confirm the fact that various types of mental impulses can have different effects on the harmony of the body and, consequently, on the individual acupuncture points. It would thus appear possible to confirm experimentally the varying types of physiological effect produced by the "*K'o*" and "*Hsi*" methods of breathing referred to in *A Thousand Ducat Prescriptions*.

Respiratory therapy is known throughout China and is practiced by many of the people. Popular scientific newspaper articles describe the exercises and explain their physiological associations and their preventive role against illness. Generally speaking, the method is extremely effective in the case of disorders of the respiratory and digestive systems and the varying forms of neurasthenia. The old Chinese writers refer to other fields of application as well, but these areas still require further testing.

On the other hand, all the traditional medical writers agree unanimously that breathing exercises cannot cure infectious diseases, poisoning, or mental illnesses.

Respiratory therapy is often used in combination with remedial massage, physiotherapy, or other traditional methods.

EFFECT ON REFLEX FUNCTIONS

It is a well-known fact that the internal organs act in a reflex manner, that is to say, that they are not controlled consciously or by the will. Yet traditional doctors in China now share the view of the historical medical works that the functions of these organs can in fact be influenced consciously and by the will with the help of breathing exercises—a practice also advocated in Indian yoga.

The Training and Research Section for Respiratory Therapy in the First Medical Academy in Shanghai carried out experiments with a man who claimed to be able to regulate pulse and blood pressure by means of breathing exercises. These exercises took the following form.[197]

The subject's blood pressure was measured on the artery of the upper arm (*arteria brachialis*). As a result of breathing exercises the *systolic* blood pressure rose spontaneously from 132 mm. Hg. to 180 mm. Hg. At the same time the *diastolic* blood pressure also increased.

The pressure sank relatively slowly during the restitution

phase; 5 to 10 minutes were required to bring it completely back to its original state. When the process was repeated several times the increase in pressure was no longer as great as that attained during the first experiment. This was only possible again after a rest period of about an hour.

The increase in blood pressure was accompanied by a heightening tension of the subject's arm musculature, although this did not extend over the whole area. This phenomenon was described by the subject as a "natural" one.

During this arbitrary alteration in pulse frequency and strength, two self-contradicting occurrences were noted—first, that the pulse increased its frequency and became strong as the blood-pressure rose, and second, that, again as the blood-pressure rose, the pulse frequency, far from increasing, actually lessened. When blood pressure increased, the pulse beat extremely strongly; when blood pressure decreased, it became very weak.

An examination of the subject's diaphragmatic breathing and size of abdomen revealed that he never remained in the exhaled state for any length of time when he wanted to increase his blood pressure. When he exhaled, his abdomen became smaller; when it inhaled, it became larger. When blood pressure increased, the abdomen decreased in size; this decrease was more clearly noticeable during exhalation than during inhalation. The Chinese researchers added the following explanation to these observations:

(a) Man can consciously influence the functioning of the internal organs with the aid of certain exercises. Such control can be developed in stages. As the above investigations show, even the function of the heart and the blood-vessel system can be controlled independently of one another.

(b) The relationship between the respiratory cycle of this male subject and the tonicity of the blood vessels runs contrary to general experience, according to which the smooth musculature of the vessels contracts when breath is exhaled and expands when breath is inhaled.

151

7

REMEDIAL MASSAGE

MAN's original medical tool is his hand, which he has always instinctively used in order to alleviate pain. Whenever he is struck, stung, or seized with cramp, he involuntarily puts his hand to the painful spot in order to protect it or to rub, knead, or massage it. The conscious use of these reflex movements can safely be assumed to date from time immemorial. In China it was obviously realized from very early on that massage not only helped to relieve pain, that is to say, that its effect was merely local; it was also seen that the stimulation of certain areas of the skin could affect the internal organs. Experience over thousands of years associated remedial massage with the same acupuncture points and meridians which have already been described in the general section of this book. In this area of therapeutics, as in others, actual practice has outstripped theory, but on the other hand, as we shall see, theories have also to a certain extent hampered practice.

Remedial massage is several times mentioned as a method of treatment in medical works dating from the Han and T'ang periods; during the latter era it was taught as a subject in the medical schools. Its importance for the art of healing, however, declined from the Sung period onwards; it was considered to be insufficiently "medical." It slowly revived during the Ming period and was used both for adults and children, not always as a method of treatment on its own, but usually in combination with other procedures.[198]

According to modern publications on traditional medicine, the type of remedial massage known as *An-mo* or *T'ui-na* has the

152

advantage of not requiring either medicaments or instruments; all that is needed is the skilled touch of the therapist's hand. Massage produces its effect both by movement of the fatty tissue and by mechanical stimulation of the skin receptors. In this way the circulation of the blood can be encouraged and—to use a traditional form of expression—the *Yin-Yang* stress ratio can be equalized. Traditional writers on this subject also emphasize the effect of this method on the musculature. Remedial massage can, for example, stimulate muscular metabolism, strengthen weakened muscles, and relieve cramp. The *An-mo* method of massage ("pressing and rubbing") tonifies, whereas the *T'ui-na* type ("thrusting and rolling") has a sedative effect.

Anyone who practices remedial massage requires strong fingers as well as sound knowledge of the relevant methods. The technique of massage is generally practiced on a sack filled with rice.[199] There are also forms of massage where the therapist makes his hands supple by applying cream or oil, or where a paste made of powdered rice or white of egg is rubbed into those parts of the patient's body where treatment is to be given.

In former times the flexors were not massaged with the bare hands; instead a small porcelain spatula, specially designed for the purpose and warmed beforehand, was used. A hen's wing, dipped in hot water, was likewise occasionally employed.[200]

REMEDIAL MASSAGE FOR ADULTS

The traditional art of healing lists eight different forms of remedial massage for adults:

1. *"Thrusting"* (*T'ui*). This is carried out in stages by means of the thumb or the ball of the thumb.

(a) *"Perpendicular thrusting"* (*P'ing-t'ui*). This is done by means of one continuous movement of a finger or the ball of the thumb in a vertical direction. This is suitable for massage of the chest, lumbar region, abdomen, and limbs.

(b) *"Lateral thrusting"* (*Ts'ê-t'ui*). This is also done in one continuous movement, but in a horizontal direction, laterally. Commonly used for head and neck massage.

(c) *"Plane thrusting" (Pao-t'ui)*. This is done backwards and forwards with a planing motion. Applied to the chest and legs.

(d) *"Semi-circular-thrusting" (Ch'an-ta)*. This is done with the edge of the thumb, and the more quickly the massage is carried out, the greater the effect. This method is mainly used on the chest along the ribs and in the region of the abdomen.

2. *"Grasping" (Na)*. By this is meant a shaking or vibrating motion which is gentle at first and becomes increasingly stronger. It is used for toning the muscles and joints and can take the following forms:

(a) *"Rolling of the muscles" (Chan-chuan-fa)*. Individual muscle cords are grasped between the fingertips and rolled backwards and forwards either with a linear or circular motion. *"Rolling"* between the palms of the hands, for example on the forearm, is also possible. This is used for the extremities only.

(b) *"Shrinking" (Chin-so-na)*. This consists of compressing the skin and muscles on the neck and shoulders into folds.

(c) *"Shaking" (Yao-fa)*. Individual muscle cords are grasped between the finger tips and shaken vigorously backwards and forwards. This is used for the limbs and in the region of the neck and sacrum.

(d) *"Vibrating" (Tou-fa)*. This consists of pressing the fingertips on the skin and moving them gently and rhythmically to and fro. Used on the limbs.

3. *"Pressing" (An)*. This is carried out either with the whole palm of the hand or at various points on the desired part of the body with the fingertips. The pressure can be gentle, medium, or very strong. There are the following methods:

(a) *"Pressing with the fingers" (Chih-an)*. This consists of exerting medium to strong pressure with two or three fingertips simultaneously. Used for the head, neck, and lumbar regions, and for the legs.

(b) *"Pressing with the palm of the hand" (Ch'ang-an)*. This is used in the abdominal region.

(c) *"Thrusting with the tip of the thumb" (Tien-an)*, supported, if need be, by the index and middle fingers, is

154

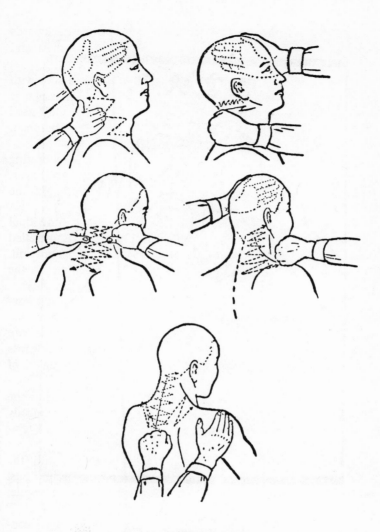

FIGURE 35
SOME OF THE MASSAGE MOVEMENTS IN THE REGION OF THE NECK
AND SPINAL COLUMN
(From a modern Chinese book on remedial massage.)
Top left: gentle rubbing with the fingers.
Top right: gentle rubbing and pressing with the ball of the thumb.
Center left: the "pincers."
Center right: horizontal thrusting and rubbing of the neck area.
Below: thrusting and rubbing of the shoulder girdle and back.

155

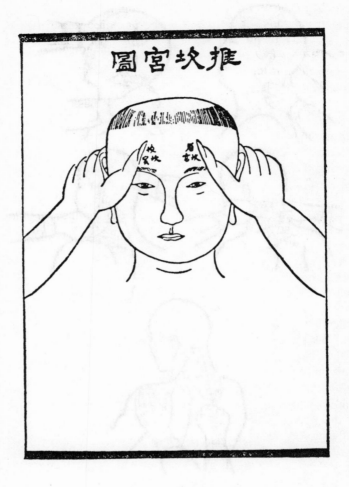

FIGURE 36
MASSAGE OF THE FOREHEAD
(From the Chinese work *Synopsis of the Technique of Remedial
Massage*, 1889.)
The Chinese caption to the picture reads: "Illustration of massage of the
K'an-kung points," the Chinese characters above the two eyebrows mean:
"*K'an-kung* points."

used at various acupuncture points. This method was already
mentioned in connection with acupuncture.

4. *"Rubbing"* (*Mo-fa*) is carried out with a quick motion, using the fingers, palm of the hand, or ball of the thumb.

5. *"Rolling with the back of the hand"* (*Kun-fa*). Here the masseur exerts gentle pressure by moving the back of his clenched fist in a rocking motion.

6. *"Pinching"* (*Nieh-fa*). This consists of grasping the skin and muscle components between the thumb and index finger or between the joints of the index and middle fingers (*"pincers"*), pressing them, releasing them and pressing them again ("as a dog bites"). This is done in the direction of the muscle fiber.

7. *"Rubbing between the palms of the hands"* (*Ch'a-fa*). This is used for the limbs and in the lumbar region.

8. *"Tapping"* (*P'o-fa*) is carried out with varying degrees of force either with one or more fingers, with the palm, side, or back of the hand, or with the fist.[201]

Gentle forms of massage tonify; strong ones, on the other hand, have a sedating effect.

The above forms of remedial massage should be used only gently with children. "Tapping" is entirely forbidden. "Thrusting" with the fingertips is not suitable for children under six years of age.[202] Special forms of massage have been developed for the treatment of children, and these are dealt with in the following section.

REMEDIAL MASSAGE FOR CHILDREN

We will now list the special forms of massage used for infants and children. These movements can, of course, also be used for adults, and will give beneficial results in the case of headaches, ear ache, sore eyes, and toothache.

1. Forms of massage for the head:
   (a) *"Thrusting into the K'an-kung points"* (*T'ui K'an-*

157

kung-fa), which are located over the eybrows. The masseur places both thumbs on the above-mentioned points and carries out a pushing movement with his left hand to the left and one with his right hand to the right. This method is effective in reducing fever.

(b) *"Thrusting into the Yin-t'ang point"* (*T'ui Yin-t'ang-fa*), which is located on the forehead above the root of the nose. This is similar to the previously described form of massage, and is of use not only for reducing fever but as a treatment for giddiness.

(c). *"Circling around the two T'ai-yang points"* (*Yün T'ai-yang-fa*), which is located in the region of the temples. The circling movement is carried out with the two thumbs simultaneously or with the tips of the outstretched fingers. According to doctors of the old school, such "circling" motion has a sedative effect if carried out in a clockwise direction and a tonifying one if done counterclockwise. This form of massage is used in cases of excessive outbursts of perspiration, high fever, and attacks of dizziness.

2. Forms of massage for the arms:

(a) *"Separation of Yin and Yang"* (*Fen Yin-yang-fa*). This consists of pushing the two *Yin* and *Yang* points near the wrist apart, using both thumbs simultaneously. This form of massage is useful in cases of shivering, bronchitis, diarrhea, and other disorders of the digestive tract.

(b) The *"eight Kua massage"* (*Yün Pa-kua-fa*) is an old term which has been retained. This form of massage consists of rubbing the palm of the hand with a circling motion from the root of the little finger to the ball of the thumb and thence back to the starting point. This has a sudorific effect and will also alleviate retching.

The *"eight Kua"* play an important part in the Taoist book of changes, the *I Ching*. They represent the eight age-old signs which have developed from the two original symbols for heaven and earth together with the combination of these two symbols in groups of three. According to the ancients, the *eight Kua* can be seen on the palm of the hand.

(c) *"Thrusting into the Shang kuan."* This consists of

158

carrying out a to-and-fro pushing motion between the *Yang-chê* point (on the wrist, beside the *arteria radialis*) and the *Ch'ü-chê* point (on the dorsal side of the elbow). If, on the other hand, massage is given from the above-mentioned *Ch'ü-chê* point towards the hand only, then this can be effective in cases of influenza, fever, bronchitis, and so on.

It is also possible to manage by stroking, starting from the

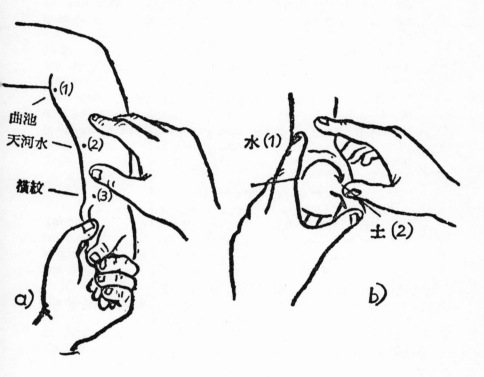

FIGURE 37
TYPES OF MASSAGE USED FOR CHILDREN
a. Massage of three points on the forearm:
   1. *Ch'ü-ch'ih* point.
   2. *T'ien-ho-shui* ("Milky Way point").
   3. Wrist flexor fold (*Hêng-wên*).
b. The method of "circling from the water element to the earth element":
   1. Direction of the water element.
   2. Direction of the earth element.

159

individual acupuncture points and leading out in various directions. Any detailed account of this method, however, would be outside the scope of this book.

(d) *"Swinging the forearm"* (*Yao Tou-chou-fa*). Here the masseur grasps the metacarpus of the child's hand with the fingers of one hand. With the other he takes a firm hold of the child's arm just above the elbow. The child's forearm is then allowed to swing gently backwards and forwards. This form of massage has a quieting effect in cases of fright and violent weeping and also stimulates the circulation of the blood.

(e) *Fei-ching Tsou-ch'i* (literally: *"the meridian flies, energy goes"*). Here the masseur gently grasps one of the child's wrists with one hand, while with the other he bends the child's fingers and at the same time presses and pinches the points on the wrist with his own fingers. According to the traditional doctors, this form of massage relieves fever and has a quietening effect in cases of eclampsia among infants. It is also helpful in cases of distension of the abdomen.

3. Forms of massage for the trunk:

(a) *"Thrusting into the Yin and Yang in the trunk"* (*T'ui-jou Fu-yin-yang-fa*). This type of massage is used in the umbilical region and is helpful in cases of diarrhea.

(b) *"Thrusting into the coccyx"* (*Jou Kuei-wei-fa*) also helps in cases of diarrhea.

(c) *"Stroking and rubbing of the Tan-t'ien point"* (*Jou-mo Tan-t'ien-fa*). This point is located a few inches below the naval; and occult significance was attributed to it in the old Taoist works. Nowadays this is the point where massage is mainly applied in cases of difficulty in urinating.

4. Forms of massage for the legs:

(a) *"Moving the legs"* (*Yao Liang-tsu-fa*). This consists of an assistant setting the child upright and holding him firmly. The masseur then grasps the child's two feet and moves his legs up and down alternately. This form of massage is also good for urinary disorders.

(b) Thrusting motions at various points on the legs.[203]

160

OLD AND NEW CONCEPTS

The concepts on which remedial massage was based changed in the course of the centuries. In olden times practical experience and interpretation were mixed with numerous superstitious elements.

Even in the sections of the "Ling Shu" there are descriptions of rational processes, albeit expressed in the language of the period. Thus, for example, in the chapters on the "healing of feverish ailments" we find that massage of certain points on the body is recommended in the case of pulmonary complaints, and that massage of the umbilical region is prescribed for abdominal pains.[204]

Later the original remedial purpose became more and more confused with irrational elements. Numerical systems were devised for the body and, in particular, for the hand. All the organs and limbs, together with everything in heaven and on earth, were incorporated in these systems. The "eight *Kua,*" which we have already mentioned, belong here as well, and were used for "reading" illness from the hand. It can thus truly be said of remedial massage that any speculation based on past history will bear scientific scrutiny only to a very limited degree. Those principles which are regarded as feasible require very thorough investigation. Empirical data, however, even if obtained without scientific explanation, have in many cases proved usable.

The old physicians also associated the fingers with the internal organs, not only as we showed when depicting the meridians, but also in a further way, namely by allotting each meridian which affected arms and legs to a certain finger joint. When one applied remedial massage, therefore, it was a case of thrusting, pressing, or rolling the finger joint associated with the diseased organ. The thumb, for example, was associated with the spleen, which belonged to the earth element, the index finger with the large intestine (metal element) and with the small intestine (fire element), and so on. In this way, practice was eventually overshadowed by speculation. The form of mas-

161

sage known as "from the water element to the earth element" reminds us of occult concepts of this kind.

According to Oriental magicians, the palm of the hand contains the secrets of life. There was also an ancient Chinese school of thought which maintained that the palm of the hand was a replica of *Yin* and *Yang* and could provide information about illness and good health and one's entire fate. Consequently, massage of the eight *Kua,* which were imprinted in circular form on the hand, could produce a cure in a "mysterious" way. The individual *Kua* are also associated with the organs; the one called *Ch'ien* symbolizes heaven, head, gold, dragon; *Tui* represents the mouth and pleasure; *K'un* is the body and earth; *Li* the eyes and the sun; *Hsün* the legs and the "broad" forehead; *Chên* the feet and restlessness; *Kên* the hands and nose; *K'an* the ears and pain.[205]

Accordingly, massage of the palm should induce harmony throughout the whole body. The massage, however, could be carried out only in a certain direction; any treatment in the wrong direction could produce a negative result. If the desired aim was not achieved, it could only be due to the "influence of some unknown element."

A sexual distinction was also made regarding massage of the hand: a man's left hand was the equivalent of a woman's right, and vice versa. Thus the true sense of the whole matter was gradually lost, and the real core of this remedial method was forced into the background.

The way in which Chinese remedial massage functions is being checked by means of modern techniques. Among other tests, for example, an investigation was carried out into the effect of remedial massage—applied centripetally and, in the other direction, centrifugally to the heart—on the circulation of the blood, the metabolic processes, and organic activity.[206]

Here the Chinese researchers are clearing away the dust of thousands of years to reveal once again the true treasures of the traditional art of healing. Thus, in the Shanghai Sanatorium for Respiratory Therapy, experiments were carried out using remedail massage as a supplementary therapeutical technique. Numerous patients were examined with the "acupuncture point micro-ammeter" in order to determine the effect of remedial massage on general physical harmony. A comparison of the results obtained before and after treatment with three arbitrary selected patients is given below.[207]

1. A 37-YEAR-OLD MAN; PROLAPSE OF THE STOMACH; MEASUREMENTS TAKEN AT FOUR POINTS:

Point	Before Treatment	After Treatment
Shang-kuan	20	15
Chung-kuan	37	21
Shên-ch'üeh	11	18
Ch'i-hai	12	17

2. A 30-YEAR-OLD MAN; STOMACH ULCER; SCLEROTIC TUBERCULOSIS:

Point	Before Treatment	After Treatment
Shang-kuan	6	40
Chung-kuan	5	45
Shên-ch'üeh	15	65
Ch'i-hai	11	47

3. A 40-YEAR-OLD MAN; NEURASTHENIA; DISTENSION OF THE ABDOMEN:

Point	Before Treatment	After Treatment
Shang-kuan	49	40
Chung-kuan	31	24
Shên-ch'üeh	35	20
Ch'i-hai	30	25

Of the three sets of results, the first shows a general evening-out, the second a sizable increase in the originally low index figures, while the third indicates a proportional lowering of all the figures—which points to a sedating effect.

8

PHYSIOTHERAPY

WE have already taken up the so-called "external exercises" in our chapter on respiratory therapy. These are intended to encourage from "outside" the state of equilibrium which the patient strives to attain from "inside" with the help of respiratory therapy and relaxation exercises.

We have noted, too, that the aims which the Taoists and Buddhists sought to attain by means of such a complex of exercises were not identical; it thus followed that there were necessarily differences in method as well, although from a historical point of view these differences belong to an earlier chapter in the long story of Chinese medicine. Originally, the development of physiotherapy was concerned mainly with matters affecting health and the care of the body, and as early as the 3rd century A.D., as we have previously observed, the well-known physician Hua T'o devoted his activities to physical culture. After observing the locomotor system of various animals, he devised exercises (*Wu-chin-hsi*) based on the movements of tigers, deer, bears, apes, and birds. Physical training and toughening exercises also proved from the very beginning to be essential for defense purposes against enemies. Thus a type of physical training with a military bias developed side by side with physiotherapy proper.

The Taoist schools of thought subsequently strove to pursue inner development (*Nei-kung*), but at the same time they taught the "external" exercises (*Tao-yin*), "in order to reach beyond the confines of the body, raise oneself beyond its restraints, and make Nature subservient to one's own power." The Buddhists, on the contrary, laid great importance on strengthening the physical constitution of the body. Bodhidharma, a famous Buddhist monk of Indian origin (6th century A.D.), laid down 18 such gymnastic exercises for monks. General Yo Fei (12th century A.D.) himself devised eight different movement exercises for his soldiers to use in attack and defense.

Thus it was that the "art of fisticuffs" (*Ch'üan-shu*) developed into a gymnastic discipline. It was not, however, anything like boxing as we know it in the West, although the exercises *are* based, as we shall show later, on forms of attack and defense. The person carrying out the exercises, however, "defends" himself in a transcendental sense and "boxes" against an "opponent" in the form of illness.

The "art of fisticuffs" dates back to two main schools, entitled *Shaolin* and *T'ai-chi*. The former derived its name from the *Shaolin* monastery in the province of Honan, where the monks had inherited the 18 toughening exercises from their abbot, Bodhidharma. In the course of time the monks developed these exercises still further, perfected them, and also taught them to other faithful believers. This school combined monastic life with the development of physical strength.

General Yo Fei and the monk Chiao Yüan also developed these exercises and built them up into a system, which eventually comprised 173 series of movements. Since the movements of the *Shaolin* school are not primarily concerned with therapy, we need not go into any further detail about them; all we need say is that they bear a certain resemblance to Japanese *karate*.

The exercises which are important from a therapeutic point of view originate from the so-called *T'ai-chi* school. *T'ai-chi* is a very old term, signifying the absolute, standing above all else. This concept of the absolute appears in two forms, *Yin* and *Yang*. According to some sources, the founder of this school of thought is said to have been Chang San-fêng (10th century A.D.), who strove to obtain complete mastery over the body by means of a combination of inward calm and movement exercises carried out slowly, loosely, and flexibly. Once physical and physiological equilibrium had been achieved, it would then be possible to repel any "assailant on the health."[208]

The *T'ai-ch'üan* exercises, that is to say, the balancing of

165

Yin and *Yang,* are not the same as the various forms of Mongolian wrestling or the Tibetan and Indian *Hatha Yoga* exercises. The term "absolute fisticuffs" must therefore be interpreted as implying that a person's mind as well as his sense organs and internal organs, together with the "harmony" of the limbs, must be in a condition of constant equilibrium. To produce such an equilibrium it is necessary to carry out slow, regular coordinated, natural, and easy movements, breathing normally all the while. The person doing these exercises contemplates his body as if its bones consist merely of a series of small "cylinders" linked together by loose joints, the whole being supported by the spinal column. The aim is to procure a condition of stability and equilibrium for this multiplicity of small "cylinders" so that they do not become disordered when the person moves or oscillate when he is jarred.[209]

BASIC THEORY OF THE EXERCISES

The principles behind Chinese physiotherapy can be summarized as follows:[210]

1. The exercises require no effort. Permanent coordination of all the limbs is achieved by concentration alone. "If the movements are angular, they must be rounded off; if they are uncoordinated, they must be coordinated. Every part of the body must be maintained in a loose and relaxed state."

2. Every movement starts from the sacral area. The "sacrum" must remain "quiet and firm." Thus Chinese authors employ a metaphor according to which the sacrum is the main shaft while the extremities are the small ones; or, if the sacrum is the large "cylinder," then the extremities are the small ones.

3. Every movement is carried out in a circular direction. Although arms and legs appear to move "angularly" in their sockets, in actual fact they describe either circles or semicircles in their swivel joints. In older times this was expressed by saying that every square contains a circle, and vice versa.

4. Equilibrium must be obtained during every phase of movement. This can be done by constantly striving to have a pre-

166

prepared center of gravity which will suit both the defense and attack positions.

5. Physiotherapeutic movements must be smooth and uninterrupted, like slow-motion pictures. The Chinese compare them to the movements of cattle chewing the cud.

6. Large weights can be moved with little expenditure of energy. The body must therefore not be tensed; on the contrary, the idea is to carry out the exercises with a continuous "momentum" and maintain the equilibrium in harmony with the constantly changing center of gravity.

7. "Strength" and "lack of strength" must be shared, which means that excess weight develops on the side of which the exerciser is leaning, and that this excess must be balanced by the "vacuum" on the other side.

8. "Upper" and "lower" must follow one another, which means that the arms and legs must be moved alternately.

9. Breathing must be deep and quiet. The shoulders must also be kept still, otherwise the person doing the exercises will begin to gasp.

10. "Movement must be peaceful and all peace contains movement." This is an alternative way of expressing the *Yin-Yang* principle and denotes "passivity in activity" and "activity in passivity." It thus follows that all movements should be reflex controlled.

According to literature on the traditional art of healing, the spiritual basis forms an essential component of the exercises. This basis includes *stamina, full concentration, continual exercising* (summer and winter, in the same way, at the same time, and as far as possible under the same conditions), and *gradual intensification.* The acquisition of a complete series of movements requires much time, since no new movement may be added until all the previous phases have been mastered. And finally, there is one more condition: the person doing the exercises must *go to bed early.*

Exercises are normally carried out in the open air, if possible in a sheltered position. The best times have proved to be half an hour after getting up and about an hour before going to bed. No heavy meals should be taken immediately before or after the exercises, and the same applies to drinking and smoking. No impeding clothing should be worn.[211]

CARRYING OUT
THE THERAPEUTIC EXERCISES

The complete series of exercises comprises some 108 movement phases, the precise number varying from author to author. During all phases the arms, legs, and head are moved in various directions with a circular motion. Old books on the subject even attached significance to the different points of the compass, but this may be disregarded. The exercises can be carried out alone or in pairs. In the latter case, two persons stand facing one another and carry out either identical or complementary movements. Thus the various forms of attack and defense are run through in slow motion, as it were. Whenever one of the participants puts his left foot forward, his opposite number likewise takes a step forward with his left foot; or, if the one partner lowers his arms, the other rotates his raised arms, so that together they form a unified motion. The exercises last approximately 20 to 25 minutes.

There is also an "advanced school" of gymnastic exercises wherein physical and mental equilibrium are combined on a higher plane. This special series of exercises is called *Ta Lü* ("the great repulse"). This means that, in cases both of actual attack or its simulation, the actor not only repels the attacker by physical force alone—he also increases the power of his bodily strength by means of the energy generated by his "calm spirit" and his steady concentration. The original source of this notion may well go back to Buddhist concentration exercises. Nowadays, *Ta Lü* exercises are regarded as a therapeutical means of achieving physical equilibrium.[212]

Chinese remedial exercises have today completely lost their

FIGURE 38
This illustration depicts 15 different movements that are to be carried out slowly, and form part of a coordinated series.

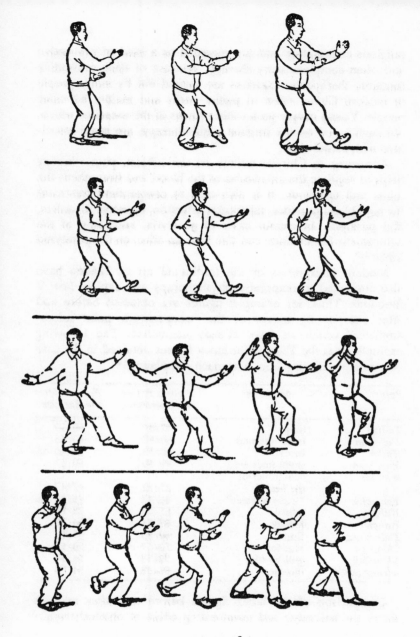

FIGURE 38
SERIES OF MOVEMENTS FROM THE T'AI-CHI-CH'ÜAN EXERCISES

religious connotation and are regarded as a kind of preventive and often complementary therapy. Because of their preventive function, therapeutic exercises are carried out by many people in modern China, often in public parks and mainly by older people. Young people prefer other forms of the exercises which, although based on the original physiotherapy, are more associated with actual sport.

According to Chinese writers on the subject, physiotherapy helps to regulate the circulation of the blood and strengthens the joints and ligaments. It is also used to complement treatment for high blood pressure, tubercular infection, digestive disorders, and paralysis. In certain cases of paralysis, exercising of the antagonistic musculature can also have an affect on the paralyzed limbs.[213]

Modern interpreters of the traditional art of healing have also attempted to reappraise physiotherapy and explain how it functions. Thus, for example, figures are obtained before and after exercise by means of the "acupuncture point micro-ammeter" which we have already mentioned. The following example gives the *Yüan* point index figures obtained in the case of a patient suffering from a stomach complaint.[214]

Point	Meridian	Figures Before the Exercise	Figures After the Exercise
Ta-ling	lung	47/52	60/60
T'ai-yüan	large intestine	60/67	63/65
Ho-ku	heart	40/53	37/40
Shên-mên	small intestine	40/50	50/57
Wan-ku	"controller of the heart"	27/52	47/47
Yang-chê	"triple warmer"	40/43	48/50
T'ai-pai	spleen	65/70	72/80
T'ai-ch'i	kidney	67/75	65/70
T'ai-ch'ung	liver	60/63	65/66
Ching-ku	bladder	50/57	50/57
Ch'iu-hsü	gall-bladder	52/53	54/54
Ch'ung-yang	stomach	53/56	54/56

Comparison of the index figures before and after exercise shows the balancing and harmonizing effect of physiotherapy.

9

OTHER HEALING PROCESSES

THE healing processes which we have thus far discussed are still commonly used in China. *Cupping,* on the other hand, is now less important.

This process has a long tradition in China. It was referred to by Ko Hung as long ago as the 4th/3rd centuries B.C. as the "horn method" (*Chio-fa*).[215] This name suggests that cupping was done with an animal's horn and not, as was the case with various other peoples of antiquity, by sucking with the mouth. The tip of a horn was cut off and the wide opening placed on the skin. The horn was then sucked till it was empty of air; the smaller opening was quickly closed and/or kept shut with one's finger. Suction then held the horn firmly onto the skin.

The horn was later replaced by cupping glasses. Modern manuals on the traditional art of healing state that, generally speaking, cupping was used only for treating the lower classes; the upper classes did not rate it particularly highly. Detailed modern works on the subject are not available, although some investigations were begun after 1949.[216]

Nowadays three different types of bell-shaped receptacles are used for cupping. One of them consists of a 6–8 cm. long and 2–4 cm. thick bamboo tube, slightly rounded at each end so as not to damage the skin and to give the tube good suction power. The two other types consist of small bell-shaped receptacles made of burnt clay and/or glass. The commonest material used today is glass.

Doctors trained in the traditional school carry out cupping as follows. Cotton wool, medicinal herbs, or paper is soaked in

171

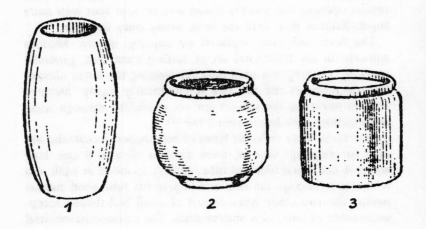

FIGURE 39
CUPPING GLASSES
Made of 1. bamboo 2. burnt clay 3. glass.

172

oil or alcohol and then burned in the cupping glass so as to warm the air inside it. When the correct degree of heat is attained, the burning material is removed from the glass. Once the doctor has ascertained that the edge of the receptacle is not too hot, the cupping glass is placed, edge downwards, on the part of the body to be treated. It remains there some 10 to 15 minutes and is then tipped over on one side and removed.

Since air contracts on cooling, this cupping process exerts a strong suction force on the skin. A small blister is produced which fills with blood. Finally, the part of the skin where treatment was applied is smeared with ointment. Formerly, the cupping glass was tipped on to the skin together with the burning material. This caused burns on the skin, and the method is no longer in use.

Besides so-called "dry-cupping" there is also "wet-cupping," which consists of scarifying the skin with a lancet-type acupuncture needle, thus enabling a considerable quantity of blood to be sucked up when the cupping process is applied. In this type of treatment the patient feels a great sense of relief. Both methods of cupping are used in the treatment of colds and rheumatic ailments, abdominal pains, diarrhea, and headaches. Contra-indications are skin diseases, abscesses, and infectious diseases. Cupping should not be used on the abdomen of pregnant women.[217]

According to a report in a Chinese medical journal, excellent results were achieved by cupping in the treatment of chronic bronchial catarrh and rheumatic ailments,[218] thus proving that it fully justifies its reputation as a method of curing.

Traditional medicine includes other disciplines, however, which are now regarded as totally out-of-date and are consequently no longer used. In the interests of medical history, however, we shall now briefly describe the more important of these.

A historical curiosity in the Chinese art of healing is the method known as "straightening the bones" (*Chêng-ku*), which contains surgical as well as orthopedic features. Bones which had slipped out of position were jerked back into place, as is the general practice today.

Attempts were also made to straighten bones which had been

173

distorted by rickets by placing them between suitably shaped boards. This method was also used in cases of curvature of the spine. Various forms of massage were applied as well.[219]

A further method of treatment is "sun therapy," known traditionally as the "*method of bearing the sun*" (*Fu Jih-mang Chih-fa*). Eventually, however, as astrological effects were attributed to the influence of the sun and other planets, all sorts of superstitions attached themselves to such therapy. For example, the patient would be handed a red or green sheet of paper containing the necessary magic formulae for collecting the sun's energy. It is difficult to find any concrete proof of success with such magic signs, but there is no doubt that sun therapy had a certain value due to the activation of vitamin D.

The concept of the world as a unity of macrocosm and microcosm regards man as representing *Yang,* that is, the sun's energy, and woman, on the other hand, as the embodiment of passive *Yin,* the moon's energy. Women were consequently exposed to the moon, not sunshine, and were handed a yellow sheet of paper on which magic signs were inscribed in Chinese ink to collect "lunar radiation."

It seems possible that such cures originated with the shamans, for in times of prolonged drought the "rain-making" witch-doctors would lie down in the full sun and attempt to convince the forces of nature to take a more reasonable view.[220]

Mention should also be made of an old Chinese custom whereby the face of a smallpox sufferer, once the disease had subsided, was covered with a red cloth, the daylight also being filtered through a red curtain. The old Chinese presumably possessed no concrete evidence regarding the harmful effects of solar radiation, yet it seems possible that this custom may well have prevented many invalids from incurring excessive pock-marks.[221]

There is also a long tradition of *hydrotherapy* in China. Wet packs and courses of treatment involving "taking the waters" were both known, as were thermal baths, mainly prescribed for rheumatic ailments. Various "miraculous springs" were also especially popular.

Any list of the various methods of cures must also include "*health by praying,*" which was once a separate branch of the

174

art of healing but which was later banned from medicine. Together with other procedures it was still mentioned in the *History of the Sung Dynasty* as late as the 14th century. Shun Hsi, who also lived during the *Sung* period, even wrote a medical work on the subject, in which he listed 13 groups of magic formulae and prayers.[222] The magic formulae include monosyllable words, described as "illness-expelling," as well as incantations in the form of requests or commands addressed to the rulers of the underworld or the realm of shades.

We have already mentioned *surgery,* which, together with anatomy, was the most backward branch of traditional Chinese medicine. The performance of operations, particularly amputations, was considerably hindered by the idea that the body, which had been received from one's parents and forefathers, had to be returned intact to one's ancestors. Although Pien Ch'üeh (5th century B.C.) had already been concerned with questions of anatomy and embryology, surgery was subsequently largely restricted to the treatment of broken bones and the opening of suppurative boils. Other not unimportant tasks included the treatment of war injuries (*Chin-tsu*), which developed during the Sung period into a separate medical discipline of its own, and castration, for there was a heavy demand for eunuchs at the Imperial court.

Since surgery was so retrograde, there was no need to develop any knowledge of anatomy, although even in ancient times there had been close links with India, where excellent surgery was performed, including, for example, rhinoplasty and abdominal operations.

In ancient China *dentistry* also belonged to a certain degree to surgery. Teeth were generally pulled by means of the bare hands alone, and as early as the 11/12 centuries A.D. amalgams were used for filling hollow ones:[223]

Finally, we should note the *"thirteen sciences,"* the name given to medicine in the *History of the Sung Dynasty.* The art of healing was divided in those days into the following branches:
1. the "science of the wind"
2. the "science of fever"
3. the "science of the pulses"
4. "gynecology"

175

5. "obstetrics"
6. "acupuncture"
7. "moxibustion"
8. "healing of the throat, mouth, and teeth"
9. the "treatment of boils"
10. the "art of straightening the bones"
11. the "treatment of bodily injuries"
12. "respiratory therapy"
13. "health by praying."[224]

This division was later extended, along with further hair-splitting theorizing, a development which reached its height during the Ming period. There were four main views during this epoch: the *Yin-Yang* school attributed illness to a lack of *Yin* energy and/or to an excess of *Yang* energy; the so-called *Wên-pu* school sought to find the cause of illness in the lack of *Yang* energy; the radical school treated the "influence of demons" and feverish illnesses with "radical" vegetable medicaments; the conservative school would have nothing but the old classical works and the commentaries on them.

10

TRADITIONAL MEDICAMENTS

ACCORDING to Confucian tradition, Shên-nung taught men the use of the plough and of medicaments. Although we now know that Shên-nung was a mythical figure, it is nevertheless certain that knowledge of medicinal herbs and medicaments generally dates back to the very earliest times in China's history. Thus we find mention of certain medicaments not only on the oracle bones but also among the very oldest literary works, such as in the *Book of Songs* (*Shih Ching*), although these books did not necessarily serve any medical purpose thereby.

Knowledge of medicinal herbs and drugs was based on popular experience and was mostly empirically accumulated and spread. But alchemy was not without its influence on the further development of medicaments, although many errors were made. Neither the "herb of eternal life" nor the "golden pill," could, it is true, guarantee immortality, but the search for it presented mankind with various usable medicaments.

The great doctor of ancient times, Pien Ch'üeh, prescribed numerous medicaments. Chang Chung-ching (2nd/3rd centuries A.D.) knew of medicaments for alleviating fever, diuretics, emetics, sedating and tonifying drugs, and anodynes. His contemporary, Hua T'o, likewise used drugs for peroral anaesthesia, although details of their composition have not come down to us.

We can get a clearer picture from the various pharmacopoeia, either from the originals which have survived or from others which were later revised. The oldest of these works is the *Pharmacopoeia of Shên-nung* (*Shên-nung Pên-ts'ao Ching*), which contains the names and descriptions of 365 different

177

medicaments, together with some guiding principles for their use. Those parts of *The Yellow Emperor's Classic of Internal Medicine* (*Huang-ti Nei-ching*) entitled "Su Wên" and "Ling Shu" also list numerous drugs in connection with the description of various ailments.

At the beginning of the 4th century A.D. an alchemist physician, Ko Hung, experimented with medicaments. Later the Taoist physician T'ao Hung-ching (5/6th centuries A.D.) compared the 365 more recent medicaments collected since the Han period with those in the *Pharmacopoeia of Shên-nung*. In the 7th century A.D. medicaments and the formulae for preparing them were again collected, and an improved edition of the *Pharmacopoeia of Shên-nung,* now listing 844 medicaments, was issued.[225]

We must also mention the great Taoist doctor Sun Szû-miao, who lived at the beginning of the Tang period and who was given the title of honor, "King of Medicaments" (*Yao-wang*). Like other doctors of his time, he, too, made a collection of the medical and pharmacological knowledge which had been handed down from the previous epoch, and complemented it with his own findings. His work, *A Thousand Ducat Prescriptions* (*Ch'ien Ching Fang*), which we have referred to several times previously, contains both popular medical prescriptions together with his own secret ones. He was the first to note the various types of soya bean (*Wu-tou, Ta-tou*) which, as we now know, contain vitamin B_1, and also the bark of the mulberry tree (*Sang-p'i*), which is prized for the same reason.[226]

The spread of printing is reflected in an increase in the number of pharmacopoeia. Thus the number of medicaments listed in the 10th to the 13th centuries A.D. rose to 1082. Li Shih-chên, the noted doctor and pharmacologist who lived towards the end of the 16th century, listed 1892 different medicaments in his *Pharmacapoeia* (*Pên-ts'ao Kang-mu*), which included material from earlier periods together with his own. This work is still of importance today, and we shall therefore now give it our fuller attention.

LI SHIH-CHÊN,
DOCTOR AND PHARMACOLOGIST

Li Shih-chên was born in what is now the province of Hupei. His grandfather had been a famous itinerant doctor, and his father, likewise a doctor, had prepared his son from an early age for the medical profession. Medical "dynasties" of this kind had numerous procedures, artifices, and prescriptions of their own which were carefully cherished as family secrets and usually handed down to the eldest son as part of his inheritance.

Hupei is particularly rich in flora and fauna, and thus the child, under the influence of his domestic background and the natural features of the countryside, began to assimilate herbal knowledge very early on. The father was pleased to note his son's keenness and encouraged his interest.

Li Shih-chên very quickly saw through the hollowness of contemporary medical practice. He felt himself instinctively drawn towards the common, simple people; he would go for long walks in the surrounding woods, collect plants, and strike up friendships with the villagers, who also regarded his father with great respect. It is thus understandable that all sorts of knowledge about medicaments and cures, known only to the common people, were imparted to him. While the Taoist magicians at the courts were concocting their potions and preparing the "drink of immortality," Li Shih-chên was acquiring valuable practical knowledge; and all that remained to do was to check it and arrange it. Under his father's guidance the young man studied all the official literature on medicine and pharmacology in order to discuss these matters as well in his subsequent great work. He formed his own opinion about the Taoist magicians: "What they say is utterly and completely confused; their theories on medicine and pharmacology are dull and ponderous, and no reliance can be placed on any of them." Elsewhere he wrote, "One person took cinnabar and still died; another swallowed 'liquid gold' and also died; neither attained eternal life."[227] Cinnabar was reckoned as one of the

179

medicaments which conferred immortality; magic powers were attributed to it because it was red like blood.

Another example: the authors of two old pharmacological works were of the opinion that mercury was not poisonous and that it formed the basic component of the elixir of life. Li Shih-chên commented as follows: "During the past six dynasties up to the present day many people have taken mercury in the hope of prolonging their lives, but many of them fell ill or even died of poisoning. The Taoist alchemists must come under severe criticism; how can pharmacological books maintain such nonsense?"[228]

At the same time that he was revising the endless mass of pharmacological literature, Li Shih-chên was himself discovering new medicaments which have remained in high esteem to this day.

These include *Ch'ang-shan* (*dichroa febrifuga* Lour.), used against malaria; the antipyretic *Huang-chin* (*scutellaria baicalensis* Georgi); *I-mu-ts'ao* (*leonurus sibiricus* L., known in England as "motherwort"), used in cases of menstrual disorders; *Jên-shên* (*panax ginscheng* Nees., the "ginseng plant"), which has a tonifying effect; the diuretic *Hsiang-yu* (*elsholtzia cristata*); *Ta-fêng-yu* (the oil of the *lucraban* kernel), used against leprosy; *Ma-huang* (*ephedra vulgaris sin.* Stapf), used against asthma; *Lei-wan* (*mylitta lapidescens* Horan.) and the betel nut (*Pin-liang*), both used against helminths; the germicide *Ta-huang* (*rheum officinale* Baill, known today as medicinal rhubarb); and *Tu-chung* (*eucomnia ulmoides* Olic.), used for regulating blood pressure.[229]

Under his medicaments he also included alcohol (*Shao-chiu*), opium (*Ya-p'ien*), wine (*P'u-t'ao-chiu*), camphor (*Chang-nao*), thorn-apple (*Man-t'o-lo, datura stramonium*), and strychnine seed (*Fan-mu-pieh, semen strychni*).[230]

It took Li Shih-chên thirty years to compile his massive *Pharmacopoeia*. In the process he analyzed 758 works, consisting of 41 old books on medicaments, 277 medical works and books of prescriptions, and 440 historical tomes. He himself collected 413 medicaments by dint of drawing on his own experience and on information culled from the common people. His *Pharmacopoeia* thus contains 1892 medicaments and their indications, composed of those already known, plus 1479 types which he analyzed and catalogued. The book did not appear until 1596, after his death.

The *Pharmacopoeia* contains 52 chapters, which in turn are divided into 16 sections and sub-sections. Of the medicaments described, 492 are of animal origin (fish, birds, mammals, man); 1094 are of vegetable origin (610 herbs, 484 trees and shrubs); 275 are obtained from metals and minerals; and, finally, 31 are "everyday articles."[231]

The book had a resounding success in China and later became known in the West as well. Translations were published in Japan in 1857 and 1929. A Polishman, Michael Boym, translated parts as early as 1659; du Halde, a Frenchman, translated the entire book into French in 1735. A Russian translation by the physician-Sinologist A. Tatarinow appeared in 1857. An abbreviated German version appeared in 1928. There are more than ten known translations from English-speaking countries.[232]

In 1960 two Soviet research workers, F. Ibragimov and W. Ibragimova, published a critical evaluation of the traditional Chinese medicaments; this was mainly based on Li Shih-chên's material.[233] This book uses chemical analysis to provide a scientific assessment of some 300 Chinese medicaments.

CLASSIFICATION AND PREPARATION OF THE MEDICAMENTS

The traditional art of healing nowadays divides medicaments into three main groups, namely, those of vegetable, animal, and mineral origin; and the first of these groups is by far the largest.

Medicaments of Vegetable Origin

The characteristic active-agent content of medicinal herbs continues to change, since it is closely linked to the various phases of vegetative growth. Content is highest when the plants are fresh, but they cannot be stored for long in such a state. The drying of medicinal herbs is consequently just as common in China as elsewhere in the world.

The roots, blossoms, leaves, seeds, and fruits of herbs are all used. The traditional art of healing knew how to prepare medicaments using fire, water, or a combination of both. Methods of preparation by means of fire include drying, browning, roasting, and burning, and in the case of medicaments of metallic origin, smelting as well. The "watery" methods of preparation include soaking and moistening; to these belong the winning of alcoholic extracts. Among the combinations of the "fiery" and "watery" methods are boiling, steaming, and desiccating.[234]

The traditional art of healing also discriminates between medicaments of a cold and warm nature. In ancient times it was thought that illnesses of a "warm" nature should be cured by "cold" medicaments, and vice versa.[235] In addition, medicaments were also divided according to their taste—bitter, sour, salty, and sharp ones being considered suitable for the curing of different ailments. "A bitter taste has a 'hard,' 'strong' character and affects the heart; a sour taste, which influences the liver, has a 'composing' character; a sweet taste has mild qualities and affects the functioning of the spleen; the 'delicate' nature of a salty taste affects the kidneys and the urinary bladder; a sharp, 'dispersing' taste affects the lungs."[236]

This differentiation between the qualities of various tastes and their association with specific illnesses represents a notable discovery, already some thousands of years old, on the part of Chinese medicine. Many of these opinions which had been formed purely empirically have been confirmed by modern findings.

The connection between the heart and bitterness of taste may be roughly explained as follows: one of the chief symptoms of disorders of the biliary system is that the secretion of bile becomes congested and, as a result, congeals. Because of this difficulty in emptying the gall bladder some bile penetrates the blood system, and its bitter taste is felt by the tongue and the papillae of the mouth. The patient has thus a continual bitter taste in his mouth; whatever he eats and drinks also

182

tastes bitter. This irritation of the biliary ducts exerts a reflex effect on the vessels of the heart and causes attacks similar to angina pectoris. Nevertheless, the heart itself is absolutely sound, for this is essentially a case of visceral reflexes between it and the biliary system. Consequently, whenever a patient complains of attacks similar to angina pectoris and at the same time has a bitter taste in his mouth, then the chances are that the trouble lies with the gall, not the heart.

The connection between a sour taste and the liver can be explained by the fact that chronic diseases of the liver are usually accompanied by inflammation of the mucous membrane of the stomach and an excess production of acid. It is mainly the biliary capillaries inside the liver which are affected, and the disease is transmitted to the stomach. The disordered state of the biliary capillaries is due to chronic dysfunction of the hepatic cells of which their walls are formed. This category of patient always has a sour taste in his mouth, indicating a disorder of the liver.

The spleen and the pancreas can be regarded as belonging to one unified system, though indeed the ancient Chinese did not know of the pancreas as such. They were justified in regarding the two as one unit inasmuch as the symptomatology of the points on the spleen meridian includes the entire functional sphere of the pancreas as well. Western books on acupuncture often also describe this meridian as the spleen-pancreas meridian. We also know that the pancreas is, in addition, one of the main organs controlling sugar content in the body, and the direct effect of sweet food (sugar, carbohydrates) on this system is well known.

Another commonly known fact is that sufferers from kidney diseases must not eat strongly salted food. The susceptibility of such people to edema is closely bound up with the quantity of sodium and chlorine in the organism and its control.

No specific data is available on the relationship between a sharp taste and the lungs. It may be that strongly spiced food counteracts the consumptive's lack of appetite.

Apart from this last example, it is possible to show that four of the main qualities of taste have also a physiological part to play. This represents a great achievement on the part

183

of Chinese medicine throughout the years, which not only deserves recognition in itself but is a tribute to the powers of observation of the old physicians.

Our terms of reference do not, unfortunately, permit us to go into Chinese medicaments in greater detail at this juncture.

From the vast heritage of Chinese pharmacology we have selected the best-known medicinal herbs and listed them below, grouped according to their medicinal value.[237]

MEDICINAL HERBS FOR CARDIAC AND CIRCULATORY DISORDERS:

T'ien-mên-tung	*asparagus lucidus* Lindl. (a variety of asparagus)
Hsiang-chang	*cinnamomum camphora* Nees et Eberm. (camphor)
Pan-pien-lien	*lobelia chinensis* Lour. (lobelia)
P'u-ho	*mentha arvensis var. piperascens hort.* L (a variety of mint)
Chih-chu	*rhododendron sinense* Sw.
Yüan-shên	*scrophularia Oldhami* Oliv. (a variety of figwort)

DIURETICS:

Ta-suan	*allium sativum* L (garlic)
Yin-ch'ên	*artemisia capillaris* Thunb. (a variety of mugwort)
Ma-huang	*ephedra sinica* Stapf. (a variety of shrubby horsetail)
Hsü-sui-tzû	*euphorbia lathyris* L (a variety of spurge)
Ch'uan-ching-p'i	*hibiscus syriacus* L (a variety of marshmallow)
P'u-ho	*mentha arvensis var. piperascens hort.* (a variety of mint)
Sang-p'i	*morus alba* L (leaves and bark of the mulberry tree)
Ch'ê-ch'ien-tzû	*plantago major var. asiatica* Decne. (a variety of plantain)

SUDORIFICS:

Yin-ch'ên	*artemisia capillaris* Thunb. (a variety of mugwort)
Ma-huang	*ephedra sinica* Stapf. (a variety of shrubby horsetail)
P'u-kung-ying	*taraxacum officinale* Wigg. (a variety of dandelion)

HERBS FOR TREATING OPEN SORES:

Lu-huei	*aloe chinensis* Steud. (a variety of aloe)
Ch'ê-ch'ien-tzû	*plantago major var. asiat.* Decne. (a variety of plantain)

184

Chih-tzû-mien	*gardenia jasminoides* Ellis. (a variety of gardenia)

COUGH REMEDIES:

Sha-shên	*adenophora tetraphylla* (Thunb.) Fisch. (gland bellflower)
Ch'ien-hu	*angelica decursiva* (Miq.) Franch. (a variety of angelica)
Mu-po-tzû	*momordica cochinchinensis* Spreng.
Jên-shên	*panax schin-seng* Nees (ginseng root)
Kua-lou	*trichosanthes kirillowii* Maxim.

STYPTICS:

Ai-yeh	*artemisia capillaris* Thunb. (a variety of mugwort)
Lou-lu	*echinops dahuricus* Fisch.
Tan-p'i	*paeonia suffructicosa* Andr. (a variety of peony)
Huai-hua	*sophora japonica* L ("Japanese pagoda tree")
Ts'ê-po-yeh	*thuja orientalis* L (a variety of thuja)

TONIFYING HERBS:

Lu-huei	*aloe chinensis* Steud. (a variety of aloe)
Hsiang-chang	*cinnamomum camphora* Nees et Eberm. (camphor)
Fan-mu-po	*strychnos nux-vomica* L. (seed of the vomit-nut tree)

RESTORATIVES:

Hsüeh-chieh	*acorus calamus* L ("sweet flag")
Hsien-hao-ts'ao	*agrimonia eupatoria* L (burdock)
Shan-chu-yü	*cornus officinalis* Sieb. et Zucc. (Cornelian cherry)
Chung-p'u	*magnolia officinalis* Rehd. et Wils. (a variety of magnolia)
Jên-shên	*panax gin-seng* Nees. (ginseng root)
Hu-ma	*sesamum indicum* L (sesame)

SEDATING HERBS:

Ma-jên, Ta-ma	*cannabis sativa var. indica* L (a variety of hemp)
Pai-kuo, Jin-hsing	*ginkgo biloba* L (maidenhair tree)
Shêng-chiang	*zingiber officinale* Rosc (ginger)

PAIN-KILLING HERBS:

Fu-tzû, Fu-p'ien, Wu-t'ou	*aconitum Fischeri* Reichb. (aconite)
Hsüeh-chieh	*acorus calamus* L ("sweet flag")
Ma-jên, Ta-ma	*cannabis sativa var. indica* L (a variety of hemp)
Chü-hua	*chrysanthemum sinsense* Sabine. (a variety of chrysanthemum)

185

VERMICIDES:

Pin-liang	*areca catechu* L (betel nut)
Wu-yao	*lindera strychnifolia* Vill.
Ta-suan	*allium sativum* L (garlic)
Yin-ch'ên	*artemisia capillaris* Thunb. (a variety of mugwort)
Yen-ts'ao	*nicotina tabacum* L (tobacco)

ANTISEPTICS:

Pai-chieh-tzû	*sinapis arvensis* L (mustard)
Huang-ch'ang-shan	*dichroa febrifuga* Lour.
Ta-suan	*allium sativum* L (garlic)
P'u-ho	*mentha arvensis var. piperascens* hort. (a variety of mint)

ANTITOXICS:

Ma-tou-ling	*aristolochia debilis* Sieb. et Zucc. (a variety of birthwort)
Shan-chu-yü	*cornus officinalis* Sieb. et Zucc. (Cornelian Cherry)
Hu-ma	*sesamum indicum* L (sesame)

DESENSITIZING HERBS:

Fou-p'ing-ts'ao	*lemna minor* L (duckweed)
Hsia-k'u-ts'ao	*prunella vulgaris* L (selfheal)

HERBS FOR DISORDERS OF THE STOMACH AND DIGESTIVE SYSTEM:

Pi-ma	*ricinus communis* L (castor-oil plant)
Ma-ling-snu	*solanum tuberosum* L (potato)
Hsüeh-chieh	*acorus calamus* L ("sweet flag")
Lu-huei	*aloe chinensis* Steud. (a variety of aloe)
Ch'ien-hu	*angelica decursiva* (Miq.) Franch. (a variety of angelica)
Yin-ch'ên	*artemisia capillaris* Thunb. (a variety of mugwort)
Hsiang-chang	*cinnamomum camphora* Nees. et Eberm. (camphor)
Ch'ê-ch'ien-tzû	*plantago major var. asiat.* Decne. (a variety of plantain)
P'u-kung-ying	*taraxacum officinale* Wigg. (a variety of dandelion)

HERBS ENCOURAGING METABOLISM:

Kan-ts'ao	*glycirrhiza uralensis* Fisch. (a variety of liquorice root)
T'ien-mên-tung	*asparagus lucidus* Lindl. (a variety of asparagus)
Ch'ê-ch'ien-tzû	*plantago major var. asiatica* Decne. (a variety of plantain)
Chih tzû-mien	*gardenia jasminoides* Ellis. (a variety of gardenia)

186

SPASMOLYTIC HERBS:

I-i-jên	*coix lacrima-jobi* L ("Job's tears")
Ko-kên	*pueraria hirsuta* C.K. Schischk (hair grass)
Ch'uan-chiao	*zanthoxylum piperitum* DC.
Fu-tzû, Fu-p'ien,	
Wu-t'ou	*aconitum Fischeri* Reichb. (aconite)
Ch'ien-hu	*angelica decursiva* (Miq.) Franch. (a variety of angelica)
Ma-jên, Ta-ma	*cannabis sativa var. indica* L (a variety of hemp)
Tan-p'i	*paeonia suffructicosa* Andr. (a variety of peony)
P'u-ho	*mentha arvensis var. piperascens hort.* (a variety of mint)

ANTI-INFLAMMATORY HERBS:

Pan-pien-lien	*lobelia chinensis* Lour. (lobelia)
Hu-huang-lien	*picrorhiza kurroa* Royle.
Yüan-shên	*scrophularia Oldhami* Oliv. (a variety of figwort)
Hu-ma	*sesamum indicum* L (sesame)
P'u-kung-ying	*taraxacum officinale* Wigg. (a variety of dandelion)

HERBS AFFECTING THE CENTRAL NERVOUS SYSTEM:

Kou-t'êng	*nauclea rhynchophylla* Miq.
Yüan-chih	*polygala tenuifolia* Willd. (milkwort)
Yen-chieh-ts'ao	*ophiopogon japonicus* Ker. (white snake's beard)
Chü-lo	*citrus nobilis* L ("mandarin" citrus)
Chih-tzû-mien	*gardenia jasminoides* Ellis. (a variety of gardenia)

HERBS AFFECTING THE ENDOCRINE SYSTEM

Tzû-ts'ao-kên	*lithospermum erythrorhizon* Sieb. et Zucc. (gromwell)
Tan-shên	*salvia miltiorrhiza* Bunge. (a variety of sage)
Ch'ê-ch'ien-tzû	*plantago major var. asiatica* Decne. (a variety of plantain)
Tan-p'i	*paeonia suffructicosa* Andr. (a variety of peony)

HERBS USED AGAINST TUBERCULOSIS:

Sha-shên	*adenophora tetraphylla* Thunb. Fisch. (gland bellflower)
Tsao-chia	*gleditschia sinensis* Lam. (gleditsia)
Fêng-hsiang,	
Lu-lu-t'ung	*liquidampar formosana* Hence. (liquidambar)
Shan-tzû-ku	*tulipa edulis* Baker (edible tulip)

HERBS USED AGAINST KIDNEY DISEASES:

Tsê-hsieh	*alisma orientale* (G. Sam.) Juz. (water plantain)

187

Lu-tang-shên	*codonopsis pilosula* (Franch.) Nannfeldt (a variety of campanula)
P'u-ho	*mentha arvensis var. piperascens hort.* (a variety of mint)

HERBS USED AGAINST ASTHMA:

Fang-chi	*sinomenium acutum* Rehd. et Wils.
Pan-hsia	*pinellia ternata* Druce.
Ch'ien-hu	*angelica decursiva* (Miq.) Franch. (a variety of angelica)
Yin-ch'ên	*artemisia capillaris* Thunb. (a variety of mugwort)
Ma-jên, Ta-ma	*cannabis sativa var. indica* L (a variety of hemp)
Sang-p'i	*morus alba* L (mulberry leaves)
Ma-huang	*ephedra sinica,* Stapf. (a variety of shrubby horsetail)
Hu-ma	*sesamum indicum* L (sesame)
Ts'ê-po-yeh	*thuja orientalis* L (a variety of thuja)

HERBS USED AGAINST ARTERIOSCLEROSIS:

Ts'ung-pai	*allium fistulosum* L (a variety of onion)
Lu-huei	*aloe sinensis* Steud. (a variety of aloe)
Yen-chieh-ts'ao	*ophiopogon japonicus* Ker. (white snake's beard)

HERBS USED AS EXTERNAL CURE FOR CATARACT:

Tung-ch'ung-hsia-ts'ao	*cordyceps sinensis* (Berk.) Sacc.
Pai-kuo, Jin-hsing	*ginkgo biloba* L (a variety of maidenhair tree)
Shêng-chiang	*zingiber officinale* Rosc. (ginger)

This list of medicinal herbs includes only an infinitesimal part of all those described in the old and new traditional pharmacopoeiae. The book entitled *A Summary of the Traditional Chinese Art of Healing* (*Chung-i-hsüeh Kai-lun*) mentions some 500 basic medicaments of vegetable origin, while another book, by F. Ibragimov and W. Ibragimova, *The Basic Medicaments of Chinese Medicine,* describes in detail more than 300 vegetable medicaments. The traditional Chinese pharmacopoeiae also list full details of characteristic features, taste, effect, and dosage.[238]

As far as the administration of these medicaments was concerned, the old doctors issued instructions regarding the time of day and the phases of the moon, as well as of other cosmic constellations. Such detailed instructions are, of course, now disregarded, but modern biological research has nevertheless shown that life processes are also subject to biological rhythm and that the degree of efficacy of medicaments can consequently depend on the time of day, sunspot periods, seasons, and so on.[239]

Medicaments of Animal Origin

The stomach contents of the musk-ox (*Shê-hsiang, Moschus moschiferus* L.) were commonly prescribed for neurasthenia, anemia, or as a restorative. The horn of the Asian rhinoceros (*Hsi-chüeh, rhinocerus indicornus var. unicornis*) was ground or pounded to powder and used as an antidote to poisons or as a sedative in cases of encephalitis. The powdered horn from the antlers of a young stag (*Lu-chung*) was reputed to be effective against consumption, anemia, and rheumatic ailments. In addition, antelope horn, scorpions, and various kinds of snake poison (for example, the venom of the *Wu-shê* or *natrix vibakari*) are still to be found in Chinese pharmacies. Otter fat and honey, both of which are medicaments of animal origin, also belong here. In olden times the physicians also believed in the healing power of placenta, finger nails, urine, and feces, as well as that of various snails, marine animals, and shellfish. As with medicaments of vegetable or mineral origin, animal substances were administered in the form of tablets, powders, ointments, tinctures, or pills.[240]

We must also mention in this context the famous "dragon's teeth." These were the bones of pre-historic animals and were stocked by all pharmacies. The chemists obtained them mostly from farmers. Thus it came about that valuable archeological finds were repeatedly made in Chinese chemists' shops, including, for example, the first specimens of the Yin-period oracle bones and the teeth of the pre-historic *gigantopithecus* in South China.

A great deal of superstition was associated with medicaments of animal origin in particular. For that reason alone, traditional medicine in China nowadays uses very few medicaments of this kind.

189

Medicaments of Mineral Origin

Mineral substances have likewise been known in China since early times, and other chemicals were discovered by alchemists. Thus mercury was used not only in alchemists' laboratories but also in the treatment of syphilis. Sulphur in the form of an ointment was applied against scabs on the skin. Because of its ability to neutralize poisons and its favorable effect on anemia, orpiment (*Tz'û-huang*) was also used. Arsenic (*Hung-p'i*) was used for eczema, tuberculosis, and syphilis; zinc sulphate (*Liu-suan-hsin*) for bladder ailments; potassium nitrate (*P'o-shih*) as a diuretic (as was also done in Egypt, Ceylon, India, Iran, and Mexico); and alum preparations (*Pai-fan*) for inflammation, chiefly of the mouth and gums. In addition, medicaments were also prepared from gypsum (*Shih-kao*), calomel (*Ching-fên*), red lead (*Ch'ien-tan*), cinnabar (*Chang-sha*), and other substances.

Gold and silver, among metals, and amethysts and rubies, among precious stones, were used in medicine, and some of these inorganic substances still form part of the stock-in-trade of the traditional pharmacies.[241]

EXTERNAL APPLICATION
OF MEDICAMENTS

So far we have concerned ourselves mainly with the internal uses of Chinese medicaments; let us now deal briefly with their external applications. Chief among these is inhalation, whereby the patient normally inhales the vapor from an infusion of medicinal herbs or occasionally even the fumes from burnt plants. This is commonly used for disorders of the respiratory tracts and for skin diseases and women's ailments.

In the case of *bath treatment* the patient bathes in a concoction of medicinal herbs or in an extract obtained without boiling.

In the case of the so-called *Fu-yen* method, honey and wine are stirred into a powdered drug and then spread on to the affected part of the body in the form of a plaster. Garlic, which is well known as a stimulant for the skin, can be used in this way. Boils can be brought to a head by the *Fu-yen* method.

Other applications include treatment with ointments, the snuffing of drugs through the nose, plugging of the nostrils to stop nose bleeds, the insertion of a wad of medicinal herbs in the mouth, the administration of emetics, the application of medicinal plants either by injection, swabbing, or rubbing, and the use of expectorants. Finally, mention must be made of the *"ironing"* method, which consists of placing the medicinal herbs on the part of the body to be treated, covering them with a cloth, and warming them by means of an iron or a hot-water bottle. This method is mainly used for the alleviation of local pains and for rheumatic complaints.[242]

In order to increase the effect, several medicaments are often used in combination. The old physicians laid great value on good prescriptions, while many mixtures were jealously guarded among the people and handed down as family legacies. Li Shih-chên made a systematic arrangement of the 10,000 prescriptions which he was able to uncover, but his work still did not provide an over-all study. Such prescriptions as have been checked and found effective are adopted by both the modern and traditional schools of medicine in China alike. Many prescriptions are admirably suitable for the treatment of specific ailments which occur in certain climatic zones, such as malaria, leprosy, and snake bites. Many of these traditional cures turn out to be more effective than comparable modern medicaments.

Medical and pharmacological periodicals issued by both schools in China are at pains to make well-tried prescriptions available to all. An example is provided in the mixture of the roots of *paeonia albiflora* Pall., *aplotaxis auriculata* and *coptis teeta* Wall. prepared according to an old prescription, which proved more effective in the treatment of acute bacillary dysentery than did either *sulphaguanidine* or *streptomycin*.[243]

Acute tonsilitis can be cured, usually within two days, by infusions of *strobilanthes flaccidifolius* Nees., *arctium lappa* L, and *scrophularia Oldhami* Oliv.[244]

According to a report in a Chinese medical journal,[245] 99 per cent of 309 lepers were cured in nine months by the use of a traditional prescription, containing extracts from some 30 medicinal herbs, including *semen chaulmoograe, rhizoma atractylis, radix ledebouriellae, radix sophorae, cortex dictami,* and *cortex phellodendri.*

CHARMS AND SPELLS

Before we close, let us briefly discuss the magic attempts to attain "eternal life" which played such an important part in China's past.

How was "immortality" best to be achieved? Even in this respect there was a considerable diversity of opinion among the Taoist magicians. Many, for example, regarded mercury as the basis for the elixir of life. Others believed that in cinnabar they had found a substance for prolonging life. Others, again, reckoned that the "golden pill" (*Chin-tan*), obtained by "nine transmutations," would ensure "eternal life." According to Chinese mythology, the wife of Yi, Ch'ang O, had stolen a golden pill from her husband and swallowed it. Fearful of being punished, she thereupon fled to the moon, the "Great Cold Palace," where she lives to this day. According to the *Historical Records* (*Shi Chi*), which were compiled around 90 B.C., "the magician uses a fire and crucible to prepare the drink of immortality, and when he has drunk it he finds the 'Isle of the Blessed.' "[246]

Let us take a look at an alchemist's laboratory: "Water had been put into the magic furnace and coal added"—thus Shun T'i begins his account (8 A.D.)—"then the furnace was sealed and everyone went away. Some months later the seals were examined; they were found to be secure and untouched. Then the furnace doors were opened in the presence of the local mandarin and other dignitaries. The coal had burned away to ashes, which were collected and put on one side. The elixir emerged, as expected, without the help of any human agency. First of all it sent out rays in five colors, then it grew as bright as the sun and shone forth at the side of the furnace. The

192

emperor swallowed this shining pill and obtained eternal life and celestial bliss."[247]

Had the substance really changed into the "elixir of life" in the *athanor* (magic furnace)? We may well doubt it. Waley suggests that the alchemist may possibly have discovered some phosphorescent substance, perhaps a phosphorescent variety of calcium sulphide.[248]

There is also a long tradition behind the "herb of eternal life"

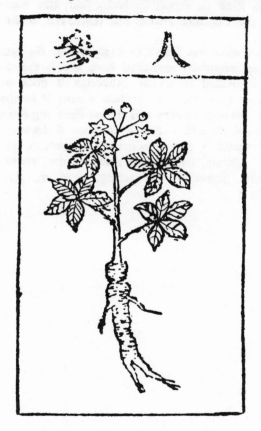

FIGURE 40
ILLUSTRATION OF THE GINSENG ROOT
(From a modern reproduction of the *Pharmacopoeia* of Li Shih-chên, 1518–1593.)

193

as well as the "elixir." There were varying views on this subject as well. Many thought that they had found the real solution in *Huang-lien* (*coptis teeta*), while others preferred *Yüan-hua* (*daphne genkwa* Sieb. et Zucc.). Most popular of all, however, was *Jên-shên,* the ginseng root (*panax gin-seng* Nees.). This root is similar to the human body; the two tips of the root are like legs and the two upper continuations of the root are like arms. It is also a very rare plant, and the mere discovery of one was in itself an especially lucky find; this was why this wonderful plant became known and celebrated as the "herb of eternal life."

Modern science has found an explanation: the ginseng root is indeed an important medicinal herb and is therefore systematically cultivated in China. Although it does not confer eternal life, it is, in fact, an excellent means of tonification for the central nervous system and a first-class regulator of high blood pressure. It is also effective in cases of diabetes. According to Ibragimov's pharmacopoeia, it contains phosphorus, potassium, calcium, magnesium, sodium, iron, aluminum, silicon, barium, strontium, manganese, titanium, glucose, and volatile oils [24]

11

FUTURE DEVELOPMENTS

WITH some justification it might be asked: What is the actual value of traditional Chinese medicine in this day and age? Many of its ideas, limited in their development by virtue of the historical times in which they were conceived, cannot be applied today without further examination. And again, can the expected result justify the years of toil involved in the requisite scientific research?

This last chapter will attempt to answer these questions, though of course we can provide only a modest survey of what is a vast and varied field. The traditional Chinese art of healing covers a huge area of knowledge, and to deal with it in detail is far beyond our present scope. Even for an expert, the acquisition of a thorough knowledge of all the various aspects would probably demand more comprehensive study than is required, by comparison, for modern medicine. Not that we intend by any means to deprecate the value of modern medical achievements. On the contrary, the traditional Chinese discoveries require examination and assessment by present-day methods. In the process there must be no attempt to justify deficiencies in the traditional views and procedures at all costs, nor must there be any attempt to see in them a deeper significance than the actual one which is immediately apparent. But any practical knowledge which is adjudged to be correct and usable should be made available to all, for there is no doubt that the traditional art of healing still conceals much of immense value.

Even prior to 1949 there were repeated reports of sensational findings, but it was only after the political revolution that systematic research truly began.

Anyone who expected a miraculous cure would often have been bitterly disappointed if, around the turn of the century or even later, he had undergone exclusively traditional courses of treatment. Let us quote, for example, from the autobiography of the President of the Chinese Academy of Science, Kuo Mo-jo, who also studied modern medicine in Japan.[250]

"My father knew something of the Chinese methods of healing," he writes, "although he was not a trained doctor. He relied on his common sense and practical experience and thus obtained considerable knowledge of medicine and medicaments. Whenever he examined a patient, he did not feel his pulse, nor did he talk about magic theories, or about *Yin* and *Yang* and the five elements. He would study the expression on the patient's face, ask him how he felt, make him show his tongue to see if it was furred, and take his temperature. There was no trained doctor in our village, so that, although my father had no sign hanging outside his door, a great number of patients came to him, the majority of whom were cured by means of the administration of medicaments. The villagers without exception revered my father as a life saver. Our uncle often teased him about it, calling him the 'great miracle doctor.'

"When I came back from abroad—I was suffering from typhoid—my father, as was his wont, prepared some pleasant-tasting medicine or other and administered it to me. Anyone who fell ill in our house was treated with one of my father's medicaments. Only this time my illness seemed to be so serious that even my father did not know what was to be done. He therefore called in the qualified Chinese doctor Sung Hsiang-chên, who lived in the next village.

"Dr. Sung Hsiang-chên was a *Hsiu-ts'ai* (meaning 'outstandingly gifted'—a title which was obtained in pre-revolutionary China by taking an official local examination). He was not a local man, but came from Liuhuahsi. I knew that he was an orphan and that he had come to work as an assistant in a chemist's shop. The chemist noted that his assistant had good powers of observation, and took him on as an apprentice. He

196

taught him to read, and then his real training began. He later married the chemist's daughter. It was thus only natural that Sung should now earn his daily bread by practicing the art of healing. His medical reputation was based, as he himself put it, less on his expert knowledge than on his place in the scientific hierarchy ensured by his *Hsiu-ts'ai* title. The villagers did not like to go to him—possibly because they were afraid he might charge too much.

"My father was a close friend of Sung's, and, although he had no great confidence in his ability as a doctor, he nevertheless consulted him about my serious illness in order to have an expert's opinion.

"As regards the diarrhea I was suffering from, Dr. Sung said it was a *Yin* ailment; in his opinion the fever, nose bleeding, and other symptoms were 'external' ones. The first thing to do was to cure the 'internal' ailment, then the 'external' ones. He also supplied a prescription and the drugs for medicine. The diagnosis was made on the second day following my return home. The fever then went down a little, which was a perfectly natural thing for it to do, as in typhoid cases it is always lower in the forenoon and higher again in the afternoon. On the previous evening I lost consciousness; my temperature must have risen to over 104°. My aunt boiled the medicine which had been prescribed. My uncle also tended me, and while the medicine was being boiled he kept advising my aunt not to let it boil over and yet at the same time to make it very thick.

"I had to drink down a large receptacle filled with this hot and viscous medicine. Scarcely had I done so than I began to feel the effect. All mucous membrane turned dark, and there was not a single bright speck left on the membrane of my mouth, tongue, eyes, and nose. At the same time inflammation started up in my lungs. I cried out, like a madman: 'I want to lie down on the ground! I want to lie down on the ground!' I no longer wished to lie quietly on my bed, and I kept trying to get down on to the floor. Even when I lost consciousness I kept shouting to be laid down on the ground. Everyone who heard me was alarmed, and the whole family was terrified. Dr.

Sung stood there just as helpless as my father and uncle. It was obviously too late to fetch another doctor from the town since the patient would probably be dead before he arrived.

"For the time being, however, it was too soon to speak of dying, for I was still breathing. But something had to be done, so a magician was sent for to drive out the devil. I was told later that a cock was killed at my bedside and its heart cut out and placed on *my* heart—for what reason I know not. I was then given all sorts of pills. Everything was tried.

"On the forenoon of the third day my uncle fetched a doctor called Chao. Dr. Chao lived on the other side of the river in Taiping, some 30 li (about 15 kilometers) away. We had never heard of him before. My uncle, who brought him, had got to know him quite casually, but, acting on the assumption that in an emergency it is better to do something rather than nothing, he seized the opportunity and went and fetched him. There was no other solution but to try Dr. Chao. He arrived on the forenoon of the fourth day. No sooner was he there than the battle began, for Chao was of the exact opposite opinion to Sung. He maintained my illness was a *Yang* one and required cold medicine. He also supplied a prescription together with the ingredients (sodium sulphate and rhubarb). I need not tell you that Dr. Sung disagreed. Nor could my father bring himself to support this new proposal. The arguments flew backwards and forwards. They debated the matter all forenoon and all afternoon. I think five o'clock came, and they still could not decide which course to adopt. My mother eventually lost patience and went in to demand a decision.

"When my mother came to see to me for the last time, it was already growing dark. Only my sister was sharing the vigil with me, and I was already half dead. My darkened mouth was wide open and my eyes were rolling. When I lay still, I looked like a corpse; when I was restless, I flailed about like a madman.

"Dr. Chao was very confident and insisted in principle on his method. He said that if we did not do as he said he might as well go. Although, he said, his medicine contained an aperient, the patient's diarrhea would diminish from day to day until he was completely 'dried out.' He would not agree to my father's proposal to reduce the prescribed dosage slightly. People said

198

afterwards that Dr. Chao had rarely been so decisive as then.

"My behavior was strange enough in all conscience, which led my mother to believe that the demons did not want to let me die, for, obviously unconscious, I kept calling out: 'I want Chao's medicine!'

"To everyone's surprise, once I *had* taken his medicine, my condition stopped deteriorating and the diarrhea began to subside. According to the doctor's instructions, I had to continue to take the medicine. He had prescribed six doses, one every second day, if I remember rightly. Two weeks passed in this fashion, and I now passed a black stool with a pungent odor. I slowly regained consciousness and became aware of the smell. According to the doctor's orders I still had more of the medicine to take, but my father held other views and prepared a potion of his own, which he administered to me.

"Possibly I was not destined to die of typhoid; on the other hand it is possible that my father saved me, for after typhoid fever the intestine is easily perforated. When the internal scabs work loose, the scars which are left bleed very easily. To administer aperients during this phase of the illness can therefore have catastrophic results.

"Gradually my high fever subsided. Some three weeks had passed without my eating or drinking. I grew so thin that I was nothing but skin and bone. A further three to four weeks passed before I could sit up and remain seated without swaying. Unfortunately there were complications. I lost my hearing for a long time, and to this day it is poor—the result of inflammation of the middle ear caused by the typhoid fever."

Our object in quoting this account is to illustrate the state of health service in a Chinese village around the turn of the century. There was utter confusion between superstition and serious practical experience and the two had become inextricably bound up together. This state of affairs changed very little up to the time of the political revolution. It is true that doctors who had received modern training ignored the traditional art of healing, but they were unable to raise medical standards in any other way.

Thus the political upheaval brought a significant change in the field of public health. A start was made in spreading mod-

199

ern medical knowledge on a broad basis. Nevertheless, in relation to the vast amount of territory and China's huge population, the number of doctors with modern training remains a very modest one. For the time being, the only solution to the problem of providing medical care for the population lies in cooperation between the modern and traditional doctors.

During the struggle against the Japanese, and also during the Civil War, there was great difficulty in providing both soldiers and civilians with modern medicaments and medical care. Recourse was therefore had to those traditional methods of treatment which were well-tried and had proved effective; in many cases they yielded better results than modern methods did, and they required no expensive medicaments.

After the Civil War came to an end, the People's Government called upon all doctors to make a systematic study of the traditional medical methods. Thus it was that thousands of doctors who had had a modern training also learned about the traditional processes.

Yang Fu-chi, for example, carried out highly successful work in the province of Hupei. An article about his work and achievements[251] states that "he mastered the old Chinese art of healing by means of acupuncture." Between 1956 and 1958 he treated 146 deaf mutes with this newly acquired method. The results achieved were quite promising, for after treatment the majority of his patients were able to hear the ticking of a clock and to say sentences of three to five words as well as answer simple questions. Yang then began investigating why the treatment was only partially successful; he concentrated his research on the back of the head, on the so-called *Ya-mên,* which means roughly "silent point," where the needle is applied. Traditional acupuncture literature recommends that at this point the needle should not be inserted more than "four-tenths of an inch" in order to avoid complications.

Yang Fu-chi carried out his investigations on the assumption that the lack of success was due to the fact that the treatment was not carried out at sufficient depth in the area of the "silent point." He came to the conclusion that the reason for the warning regarding too deep an insertion was the fact that this point on the body is surrounded by a large number of blood vessels. From this he concluded that a deeper penetration could be risked only if the needle were inserted with the maximum accuracy. He had the first experiment carried out on his own person, the needle being inserted to a depth of one-and-a-half inches. After this treatment numerous patients were able to hear and, consequently, speak much better.

Yang then combined acupuncture with electrotherapy. The effect of this newly developed method on, for example, a patient such as Liang Chun-yang was so successful that after one single treatment session he regained the power of speech which he had previously lost as the result of a cerebral hemorrhage. Even a 15-day course of simple acupuncture treatment had failed here.

A further decisive step as regards future development was the setting up in 1955 of the Traditional Chinese Medical Academy in Peking and, as part of it, the Research Center for Acupuncture and Moxibustion.[252] Subsequently, the government kept calling on both modern and traditional doctors to cooperate more and more closely. In 1959 a 16-day national conference of doctors was held in Paoting, at which demonstrations were given of methods adopted and results achieved by traditional medicine. Courses with a similar content were held in individual towns and provinces, each one being attended by 70 to 80 doctors who had had modern medical training and who had already been practicing for several years. In this way some 2000 modern doctors went through these courses.[253]

In numerous new hospitals scientifically trained doctors are working side by side with colleagues who learned in the old traditional way. Since 1955 more than 300 hospitals and clinics have been set up for the use of traditional medical methods. Nevertheless, traditionally trained doctors also attend courses to make themselves familiar with modern medical methods of treatment and to equip themselves to cope with the medico-political tasks facing their great country. As an example: between 1956 and 1958, in the battle against malaria, 134,000 patients were cured by means of traditional methods.[254]

In order to encourage the spread of knowledge of traditional medicine, 13 academies and many hundreds of technical schools were set up between 1955 and 1959; at these in-

201

stitutes some 7000 students study both the traditional methods and the basic principles of modern medicine. The collection, annotation, and re-publication of old medical and pharmacological works is also proceeding apace, as we have already noted.

Many features of the traditional art of healing reflect conditions which are peculiarly Chinese. In the original primitive community both in feudal and semi-colonial China the inhabitants were left to their own resources. The lack of any formal medical service forced people to look after their health themselves, and in many cases their only recourse was to their own practical experience or to whatever had been handed down to them. That is why there are, to this day, people who are not professional doctors but who know something about the treatment of certain illnesses. They have a vast store of knowledge, albeit of an exclusively practical kind, concerning certain methods of treatment. A record is consequently kept in China of all such amateur practitioners, together with their traditional prescriptions and methods of treatment. Thus in the province of Hopei, for example, between 1955 and 1959 some 1800 of such traditional non-medical practitioners were officially recognized. This figure gives some indication of the vast number involved.[255]

Ever since the collection of these "secret" processes began, Chinese from all levels of society, from doctors of the old school down to peasants, have been passing on any prescriptions and medical methods they know. These are then collated and tested by scientifically trained doctors, and more than a few of them have turned out to be extraordinarily effective.

Here and there, methods of treatment came to light which were effective in the case of illnesses which could either not be dealt with at all by modern procedures or, at most, with only slight chance of success. Among these are arthritis, chronic nephritis, high blood pressure, poliomyelitis, and leprosy. The treatment of appendicitis without surgery is also a widespread and highly successful technique. Chinese literature even contains references to the complete curing of malignant tumors.[256]

The collection of "popular" prescriptions has also been

highly successful. In 1958 some 162,000 were collected in the province of Hopei alone. In the Shihchiachuang hospital (Hopei province), for example, epidemic brain fever, type "B" (*encephalitis epidemica*), was treated by the use of traditional prescriptions and methods. The percentage of successes amounted to 95, and the Chinese Ministry of Health recommended the general introduction of the procedure.[257]

Chinese medical journals deal with the results obtained by the traditional art of healing in great detail, including such topics as "Respiratory Therapy,"[258] "The Treatment of Measles in Traditional Medicine,"[259] "Notes on the Treatment of Simple Digestive Disorders (*dyspepsia simplex*) by Means of Acupuncture,"[260] "The Combatting of Mawworms (*ascaris lumbricoides*) with the Aid of *Quisqualis indica* (*Shih-ch'iin-tzû*),"[261] "The Effect of Cupping in 21 Cases of Chronic Bronchial Catarrh and Rheumatic Complaints,"[262] and Tuberculosis Treatment and Its Place in Medical Science in Our Country [China]."[263]

In addition to what is published in the technical journals, the present-day merits of the traditional art of healing are discussed in countless newspaper articles, the main topics frequently being respiratory therapy and physiotherapy.

The Soviet Academy of Science is also taking part in this vast work, and the Soviet Union has sent various doctors to carry out research tasks in China. Professors of medicine, including W. G. Wogralik, E. D. Tükotschinskaja, M. K. Usova, N. M. Osipova, and others, have made a thorough study of Chinese therapeutic processes. According to I. I. Fedorov, "popular" Chinese medicine contains a vast amount of valuable practical experience which, once it has been properly checked and evaluated, could enrich the world storehouse of medical knowledge.[264]

In 1958 three members of the Chinese Medical Academy published a paper which appeared both in professional medical journals and in the daily paper *Renmin Ribao* under the title, "The Traditional Chinese Art of Healing Is a Science Which Must Be Taken Seriously."[265] This paper expounds the theory that the traditional Chinese art of healing, far from being a mere accumulation of random experiences, as it has hitherto been taken to be, is on the contrary a unique system in its own right.[266]

According to Chinese statistics for 1959,[267] the number of doctors with modern training amounts to roughly 70,000 compared with some 500,000 trained in the traditional school. This tremendous disparity is in itself enough to show how necessary it is to employ both types of doctors in the interests of public health.

* * *

Our intention in writing this book was to acquaint the reader with the theory behind the traditional art of healing and its chief methods of treatment. At the same time, we have tried to give a broad outline of the present state of research and to touch on some of the unresolved questions. The differing views held as to the merits of the various therapeutic measures also show that research work is facing decisive problems.

It is only now that China is becoming more closely acquainted with the methodics of a medical system based on scientific principles. For that reason, competent experts must, for the time being, treat any submitted data with critical reserve. We hope only to have pointed out the possible future advantages inherent in the revelation and application of a school of medical thought based on practical experience covering some thousands of years. We hope too that this book will have been of a certain amount of value inasmuch as it evaluates a great deal of Chinese source material and has taken both old and new evidence into account.

SYNOPSIS OF RESEARCH UNDER THE DIRECTION OF KIM BONG HAN

SUMMARY of the contents of a paper by Professor Kim Bong Han (Pyongyang, North Korea) on the meridian system in the human body, which appeared in the newspaper *Renmin Ribao* on December 14, 1963.

THE MERIDIAN SYSTEM

INTRODUCTION

PART I. MORPHOLOGICAL INVESTIGATION OF THE MERIDIAN SYSTEM

I. Morphology of the Bonghan Corpuscles
  1. Anatomical investigation of the Bonghan corpuscles
     (a) Anatomical investigation of the surface Bonghan corpuscles
     (b) Anatomical investigation of the deep-layer Bonghan corpuscles
  2. Histological structure of the Bonghan corpuscles
     (a) Histological structure of the surface Bonghan corpuscles
     (b) Histological structure of the deep-layer Bonghan corpuscles

2. There are two types of Bonghan ducts.
3. The Bonghan fluid circulates in the meridian system.
4. The Bonghan corpuscles display characteristic bioelectric activity.
5. The Bonghan corpuscles and ducts contain a large quantity of nucleic acid, particularly DNA (desoxyribonucleic acid).

CHRONOLOGY

DYNASTY	DATES	HISTORY OF PHILOSOPHICAL THOUGHT	POLITICAL AND SOCIAL HISTORY	ECONOMIC HISTORY	HISTORY OF MEDICINE	IMPORTANT FIGURES IN THE HISTORY OF MEDICINE
Hsia	2205–1766 (?) B.C.	Shamanism and magic.	Legendary rulers; patriarchism; village communities. Ruler referred to as "*Wang*" (king).	Primitive implements; trade by barter.	Simple empiricism; shaman doctors and magicians; medicinal herbs; oracle bones with the names of illnesses.	
Shang-Yin	1766–1122 (?) B.C.					
Chou	1122–255 B.C.	Development of the *Yin-Yang* principle and the doctrine of the five elements. Important philosophers: K'ung-tzŭ, 551–479 (?), main work *Lun-yü*; Lao-tzŭ, 4th–3rd centuries (?), main work *Tao-tê Ching*; old imperial legends.	Transitional phase between the original community forms and the society of antiquity. Emergence of warring principalities; early form of feudal system.	Trade by barter between the domains controlled by the various rulers.	Inclusion of the *Yin-Yang* principle and the *five elements* in medicine. Regional differences in methods of healing. (Shantung: stone needles. Shensi: medicinal herbs. Hopei: moxa. Hupei: metal needles. Honan: massage.) *Book of Ailments*, 3rd–2nd centuries (?).	Pien Ch'üeh, the "Father of the Pulse," 5th (?) century; Tso Chiu-ming, 5th–3rd centuries (?), the first to mention acupuncture and moxibustion.
Ch'in	255–206 B.C.	Shi Huang-ti has all books burned except the medical ones (213).	Emergence of a patrician aristocracy in the towns.	Trade concentrates at centers of communications.		Hua To, inventor of anaesthesia; Chang Chung-ching (?); Wang Shu-ho, 3rd (?) century.
Han	206–220 A.D.	Cultural links with India; awareness of Buddhism.	Patrician aristocracy in the towns seizes power.		*The Yellow Emperor's Classic of Internal Medicine*, 26 (?); *Book of Medicaments of Shên-nung* (?); *Treatise on the Various Kinds of Fever*, 2nd–3rd centuries; *Short Version of the Golden Shrine*, 2nd–3rd centuries; *Book of the Pulse*, 3rd (?) century.	

209

DYNASTY	DATES	HISTORY OF PHILOSOPHICAL THOUGHT	POLITICAL AND SOCIAL HISTORY	ECONOMIC HISTORY	HISTORY OF MEDICINE	IMPORTANT FIGURES IN THE HISTORY OF MEDICINE
Era of barbarian conquests	220–618	Intensified links to foreign countries.	Late forms of feudalism.	Patriarchal form of taxation.	Translation of great medical works. The book *Pao P'u-tzŭ*, 4th century.	Ko Hung, 4th century; T'ao Hung-ching, 5th century.
T'ang	618–907	Heyday of Buddhism; beginnings of the art of printing: *Encyclopedia of the Emperor T'ai Tsung*, 10th century.	Growth of feudal power but limited by official legislation.	Beginnings of foreign trade.	First medical school (7th century); establishment of first hospital with state support. Revision of medical books. *A Thousand Ducat Prescriptions*, 7th century.	Sun Szŭ-miao, 581–682.
Sung	960–1276	Appearance of the great encyclopedias; philosopher Chou-tzŭ (1017–1073); philosopher Chang Tsai (1020–1079). Invention of the compass.	Early forms of a monetary system.	Heyday of handicrafts and manufactures. Founding of banks and issue of bank notes. Development of merchant shipping.	Reappraisal of traditional medicine; production of a bronze figure for instructional purposes.	Wang Wei-i (who had the bronze figure cast in 1027); Liu Wan-so, 1120–1180 (?).
Yüan (Mongolians)	1280–1368	Popular national traditions gain in importance.	Mongolian oppression; the old aristocracy, composed of high civil dignitaries, perishes.	Great increases in trade between the towns and foreign countries.	Publication of the popular, traditional medical works.	
Ming	1368–1644	Rediscovery and rehabilitation of the old traditional concepts.	The empire becomes dependent on the economic power of the feudal lords. Beginnings of colonization; Portuguese in Canton (1515).	Increasing importance of foreign trade. Camphor, opium, and spices sent to Europe in large quantities.	Publication of the *Pharmacopoeia* and *The Eight Special Meridians*, both by Li Shih-chên. Introduction of smallpox vaccination. Publication of some fifty new medical works.	Li Shih-chên, 1518–1593.

210

DYNASTY	DATES	HISTORY OF PHILOSOPHICAL THOUGHT	POLITICAL AND SOCIAL HISTORY	ECONOMIC HISTORY	HISTORY OF MEDICINE	IMPORTANT FIGURES IN THE HISTORY OF MEDICINE
Ch'ing (Manchu)	1644–1911	Stagnation and intellectual decay.	Foreign domination by the Manchus and colonial powers.	China cuts herself off from foreign countries and stops all trade links. Forcible exploitation by European colonial powers.	Growth of commentaries and casuistic literature. *The Golden Mirror of the Art of Healing* (1749). During the First Opium War (1839–42) China comes into contact with European medicine.	
Republic (Min-kuo)	1911–1949	Confrontation with Western science. Intellectual ferment.	China endeavors to rid herself of colonial dominance. Japanese invasion. Revolution.	Chinese opposition to the influx of Japanese goods. Economic crisis caused by armed conflicts.	Nanking government's plan to forbid traditional medicine fails in the face of protest by Chinese doctors (1929); the traditional methods gain increasing respect in Europe.	
People's Republic (Kung-ho-kuo)	1949 onwards	Establishment of Marxism and Leninism in China; at the same time a consciousness of national traditions.	Socialization and land reform.	Beginnings of industrialization.	Examination and reappraisal of traditional medical methods. Reissues of old source material; first national hygiene conference, 1950; attempt to integrate modern and traditional healing processes.	Chu Lien.

NOTES

(SEE BIBLIOGRAPHY FOR FURTHER INFORMATION ON SOURCES REFERRED
TO BELOW.)

1. Cf. *Kurzer Abriss der chinesischen Geschichte* (Short Outline of
Chinese History), Peking, 1958. Cf. for foreign languages: Tökei-Miklós,
A kinai irodalom rövid története (History of Chinese Literature), Budapest
(Gondolat), 1960.
2. Cf. *Li-shih-shang Kan-hsiang Kan-tso-ti Jên*, pp. 89–92.
3. Cf. Hou Han-shu, *Hua T'o Chüan.*
4. Li T'ao, *The Story of Chinese Medicine*, pp. 18–22; *Chung-hua
I-hsüeh Tsa-chih*, 1954, no. 2, pp. 146–152.
5. Cf. *Li-shih-shang Kan-hsiang Kan-tso-ti Jên*, pp. 99–110.
6. *Chinese Medical Journal*, 1956, vol. 74, pp. 174–191; *Pên-ts'ao
Kang-mu*, vol. VI.
7. Cf. Chu Lien, *op. cit.*, pp. 7–9.
8. Li T'ao, *Chung-kuo I'hsüeh Fa-chan-shih Ta-kang*, 1954, no. 2.
9. Székely, *op. cit.*, p. 24; Kuo Mo-jo, *op. cit.*, p. 405.
10. Cf. Huard, *op. cit.*, p. 107
11. Wang Kui, *Li Hai Chi*, p. 20. Cf. Needham, *op. cit.*, vol. II. p.
300.
12. Cf. Needham, *op. cit.*, vol. II, p. 296.
13. Cf. *Huang-ti Su-wên*, chaps. 1, 2, 5.
14. Cf. *Pao P'u-tzû*, chap. 18.
15. Cf. *Huang-ti Su-wên*, chaps. 1, 2, 5.
16. Cf. *Hsi-i Hsüeh-hsi Chung-i Lun-wên Hsüan-chi*, p. 13; Wogralik-
Wjasmenski, *op. cit.*, pp. 40–43.
17. Cf. Needham, *op. cit.*, vol. II, p. 244.
18. Cf. Needham, *op. cit.*, vol. II, p. 244.
18. Cf. *ibid.*, p. 243.
19. *Huang-ti Su-wên*, chaps. 1, 2, 5, 6, 7.
20. *Chung-i-hsüeh Kai-lun*, p. 21; Wogralik-Wjasmenski, *op. cit.*, pp.
43–48.
21. *Chung-i-hsüeh Kai-lun*, p. 21.
22. Cf. *ibid.*, p. 12.
23. Kuo Mo-jo, *op. cit.*, p. 405.
24. Cf. *Hsi-i Hsüeh-hsi Chung-i Lun-wên Hsüan-chi*, p. 20.
25. Cf. *ibid.*, p. 13.
26. *Huang-ti Ling-shu*, chap. 5.

27. Cf. *Huang-ti Su-wên.* chaps. 2. 3.
28. Cf. *ibid.*
29. *Ibid.*, chap. 10.
30. Cf. *Huang-ti Ling-shu,* chap. 77.
31. Cf. Ábrahám-Bende-Megyeri, *op. cit.,* p. 495.
32. Cf. *Chung-i-hsüeh Kai-lun,* pp. 141–144.
33. Cf. Kérdo István, *op. cit.,* p. 96.
34. Cf. *ibid.,* p. 97.
35. Cf. *ibid.,* p. 98.
36. Cf. *Wei Chih,* chap. 8, pp. 22 f.
37. Cf. *Chien-i Chên-chiu-hsüeh,* pp. 1–2.
38. Cf. *ibid.*
39. Cf. Chu Lien, *op. cit.,* p. 29.
40. Cf. *ibid.*
41. *Chên-chiu-hsüeh,* p. 88.
42. Cf. Chu Lien, *op. cit.,* p. 29.
43. *Chung-kuo Shou-i-hsüeh Tsa-chih,* 1958, no. 10, p. 492.
44. Cf. Bachmann, *op. cit.,* p. 31.
45. *Chung-i-hsüeh Kai-lun,* p. 83.
46. Soulié de Morant, *op. cit.,* p. 16.
47. Chamfrault, *op. cit.,* vol. I, p. 56.
48. Cf. Bachmann, *op. cit.,* p. 50.
49. Cf. *Chung-i-hsüeh Kai-lun,* p. 417; *Chên-chiu-hsüeh,* p. 79; Wogralik-Wjasmenski, *op. cit.,* pp. 56–60.
50. Bachmann, *op. cit.,* p. 55.
51. *Ibid.*
52. *Ibid.*
53. *Chung-i-hsüeh Kai-lun,* p. 417; *Chên-chiu-hsüeh,* p. 79.
54. Chu Lien, *op. cit.,* p. 24; *Chung-i-hsüeh Kai-lun,* pp. 417–418.
55. Cf. *Chên-chiu-hsüeh,* p. 330; Bachmann, *op. cit.,* pp. 60–61.
56. Bachmann, *op. cit.,* p. 63.
57. Cf. *Chên-chiu-hsüeh,* pp. 287–289; Bachmann, *op. cit.,* pp. 70–71.
58. Cf. *Chên-chiu-hsüeh,* pp. 17–18; *Chung-i-hsüeh Kai-lun,* p. 88.
59. Cf. *Chên-chiu-hsüeh,* p. 25; *Chung-i-hsüeh Kai-lun,* p. 93.
60. Cf. *Chên-chiu-hsüeh,* p. 33; *Chung-i-hsüeh Kai-lun,* p. 100; Bachmann, *op. cit.,* p. 150.
61. Cf. *Chên-chiu-hsüeh,* p. 27; *Chung-i-hsüeh Kai-lun,* p. 93.
62. Cf. *Chên-chiu-hsüeh,* p. 35; *Chung-i-hsüeh Kai-lun,* p. 101.
63. Cf. *Chên-chiu-hsüeh,* p. 19; *Chung-i-hsüeh Kai-lun,* p. 88.
64. Cf. *Chên-chiu-hsüeh,* p. 23; *Chung-i-hsüeh Kai-lun,* p. 93.
65. Bachmann, *op. cit.,* p. 224.
66. Cf. *Chên-chiu-hsüeh,* p. 31; *Chung-i-hsüeh Kai-lun,* p. 97.
67. Cf. *Chên-chiu-hsüeh,* p. 39; *Chung-i-hsüeh Kai-lun,* p. 105.
68. Cf. *Chên-chiu-hsüeh,* p. 29; *Chung-i-hsüeh Kai-lun,* p. 97.
69. Cf. *Chên-chiu-hsüeh,* p. 37; *Chung-i-hsüeh Kai-lun,* p. 101.
70. Cf. *Chên-chiu-hsüeh,* p. 21; *Chung-i-hsüeh Kai-lun,* p. 90.
71. Cf. *Chên-chiu-hsüeh,* p. 8.
72. Cf. Hsieh Kuan, *op. cit.,* p. 1507. Similar references in "Su Wên," chaps. 2 and 60, and in "Ling Shu," chap. 2.
73. Bachmann, *op. cit.,* p. 75.
74. Cf. Chamfrault, *op. cit.,* vol. 1, p. 617.
75. *Chung-i-hsüeh Kai-lun,* pp. 105–106.

76. Cf. Bachmann, *op. cit.*, p. 76.
77. Cf. *Chên-chiu-hsüeh*, p. 41: *Chung-i-hsüeh Kai-lun*, pp. 105–106.
78. *Chên-chiu-hsüeh*, p. 43.
79. Cf. *Chung-i-hsüeh Kai-lun*, pp. 105–113.
80. *Chên-chiu-hsüeh*, pp. 241–253.
81. Cf. Chu Lien, *op. cit.*, p. 337; Wogralik, *op. cit.*, pp. 119–160.
82. Cf. Chamfrault, *op. cit.*, vol. I, pp. 589–654.
83. *Chên-chiu-hsüeh*, pp. 11–12.
84. *Chên-chiu-hsüeh*, pp. 64–66.
85. *Chung-i-hsüeh Kai-lun*, pp. 114–118; *Chên-chiu-hsüeh*, pp. 14–17.
86. Dealt with in detail in *Chung-i-hsüeh Kai-lun*, pp. 118–135, including illustrations.
87. As, for example, in *Chung-i-hsüeh Kai-lun*, pp. 135–140.
88. Cf. Bachmann, *op. cit.*, pp. 66–68 and 252–257.
89. Cf. Huard, *op. cit.*, pp. 49–50; Wogralik-Wjasmenski, *op. cit.*, pp. 61–62.
90. Cf. Huard, *op. cit.*, p. 50.
91. Cf. *Nauka I Schizni* (Science and Life), Moscow, 1960, no. 12; Wogralik-Wjasmenski, *op. cit.*, pp. 135–191.
92. Cf. Bachmann, *op. cit.*, p. 33.
93. *Ibid.*
94. Cf. Abrahám-Bende-Megyeri, *op. cit.*, pp. 435–439.
95. Bachmann, *op. cit.*, p. 20.
96. Cf. *ibid.*, p. 26.
97. Cf. *ibid.*, p. 25.
98. Cf. *ibid.*
99. Cf. *ibid.*, p. 21.
100. Cf. *ibid.*
101. Cf. *ibid.*, p. 20.
102. Cf. Huard-Ming Wong, *op. cit.*, p. 166.
103. Cf. Abrahám-Bende-Megyeri, *op. cit.*, pp. 421–422.
104. Chu Lien, *op. cit.*, p. 24.
105. Cf. *ibid.*, p. 2.
106. Cf. Wang Hsüeh-tai, *op. cit.*, p. 9.
107. Cf. Wogralik-Wjasmenski, *op. cit.*, pp. 135–191; Ingamdschanov, *op. cit.*, p. 5; Fedorov, *op. cit.*, p. 19.
108. Cf. *Huang-ti Nei-ching Su-wên I-shih*, chaps. 17–19.
109. Cf. *Huang-ti Ling-shu*, chaps. 5, 17.
110. Cf. Abrahám-Bende-Megyeri, *op. cit.*, p. 194.
111. Cf. *Chung-i-hsüeh Kai-lun*, pp. 197–206.
112. Cf. Bachmann, *op. cit.*, p. 72; Wogralik-Wjasmenski, *op. cit.*, p. 47; Wogralik, *op. cit.*, pp. 76–85.
113. Cf. Bachmann, *op. cit.*, p. 22; *Chên-chiu-hsüeh Chiang-i*, pp. 28 f.
114. Cf. Bachmann, *op. cit.*, p. 22.
115. Cf. Stiefvater, *Was ist Akupunktur? Wie wirkt Akupunktur?* p. 10.
116. *Chung-i-hsüeh Kai-lun*, pp. 141–151.
117. Cf. *Huang-ti Nei-ching Su-wên I-shih*, chap. 42.
118. Cf. *Huang-ti Ling-shu*, chap. 20.
119. Li T'ao, *Chung-kuo I-hsüeh Fa-chan-shih Ta-kang*, pp. 146–152.
120. *Huang-ti Ling-shu*, chap. 8.
121. Cf. *Huang-ti Nei-ching Su-wên I-shih*, chap. 39.

214

122. Cf. *ibid.*, chap. 73.
123. Cf. *Chung-i-hsüeh Kai-lun*, pp. 146–148.
124. *Huang-ti Nei-ching Su-wên I-shih*, chap. 39; *Chung-i-hsüeh Kai-lun*, pp. 148–149.
125. *Huang-ti Ling-shu*, chap. 4.
126. Cf. *Chung-i-hsüeh Kai-lun*, p. 149.
127. Cf. *ibid.*
128. *Ibid.*, p. 150.
129. Cf. *ibid.*, pp. 150–151.
130. *Ibid.*, p. 151.
131. *Huang-ti Nei-ching Su-wên I-shih*, chap. 47.
132. *Chung-i-hsüeh Kai-lun*, p. 175.
133. Cf. *ibid.*, pp. 152–172.
134. Cf. *ibid.*, pp. 182–207; Wogralik, *op. cit.*, pp. 73–85.
135. Cf. *Chung-i-hsüeh Kai-lun*, pp. 212–224.
136. Cf. Huard-Ming Wong, *op. cit.*, p. 21.
137. Cf. Bachmann, *op. cit.*, p. 57.
138. Cf. *Huang-ti Ling-shu*, chaps. 9, 55; *Chung-i-hsüeh Kai-lun*, pp. 401–409; *Chên-chiu-hsüeh*, pp. 268–274.
139. Cf. *Chung-i-hsüeh Kai-lun*, pp. 379–390.
140. *Chên-chiu Ju-mên*, pp. 47–50.
141. Cf. Chu Lien, *op. cit.*, p. 35.
142. Cf. *ibid.*, pp. 16, 24.
143. Cf. *ibid.*, p. 16.
144. Cf. *ibid.*, p. 25.
145. Cf. *ibid.*, pp. 11, 24, 116.
146. Cf. Wang Hsüeh-tai, *op. cit.*, pp. 8–12.
147. Chu Lien, *op. cit.*, pp. 36–37.
148. Cf. *ibid.*, pp. 3–5; *Chên-chiu Ju-mên*, pp. 3–4.
149. Chu Lien, *op. cit.*, pp. 339–345.
150. Cf. *Hsin-pien Chên-chiu-hsüeh*, statistical table.
151. Cf. *Chung-hua I-hsüeh Tsa-chih*, November 1956.
152. Cf. *Chinese Medical Journal*, vol. 75, no. 2 (1956), p. 202.
153. *Huang Chia-ssu*, *op. cit.*, p. 24; *Chung-i-yao Tsa-chih*, February 1957.
154. Cf. Wogralik-Wjasmenski, *op. cit.*, pp. 301–313 and bibliography; Ingamdschanov, *op. cit.*, pp. 123–138.
155. Karl Baunscheidt, *A Baunscheidtismus* (Baunscheidtism), edited by Bába Imre, Szeged, 1865.
156. *Ibid.*, p. 20.
157. Cf. Huard-Ming Wong, *op. cit.*, pp. 166–167; *Chien-i Chên-chiu-hsüeh*, pp. 1–2.
158. Cf. Huard-Ming Wong, *op. cit.*, pp. 166–167.
159. Cf. *Chung-i-hsüeh Kai-lun*, pp. 411–412.
160. Cf. Chu Lien, *op. cit.*, pp. 74–75.
161. Cf. *Chên-chiu Ju-mên*, pp. 55–56.
162. As, for example, in *Chung-i-hsüeh Kai-lun*, p. 412.
163. Cf. Wang Hsüeh-tai, *op. cit.*, p. 8.
164. Wilhelm Helmut: A Chou Inscription on the Technique of Breathing. Quoted by Needham, *op. cit.*, vol. II, p. 143.
165. Cf. Ch'ên Tao, *op. cit.*, p. 3.
166. As, for example, in *Huang-ti Su-wên*, chaps. 1, 2, 8.

215

167. Cf. Needham, *op. cit.*, vol. II, p. 144.
168. Cf. Ch'ên Tao, *op. cit.*, p. 3.
169. Cf. *Hsi Ching Tsa-chih*, chap. 3: Needham, *op. cit.*, vol. II, p. 83.
170. Ch'ên T'ao, *op. cit.*, pp. 1–2.
171. *Ibid.*, pp. 1–6.
172. Cf. *ibid.*
173. Cf. *ibid.*
174. Cf. *Ch'i-kung-liao-fa Chiang-i*, pp. 3–6.
175. *Chung-i-hsüeh Kai-lun*, pp. 542–543; *Ch'i-kung-liao-fa Chiang-i* pp. 16–18.
176. Cf. *Ch'i-kung-liao-fa Chiang-i*, pp. 10–14.
177. Cf. *ibid.*, pp. 14–15.
178. Cf. *Chung-i-hsüeh Kai-lun*, pp. 545–549; *Ch'i-kung-liao-fa Chiang-i*, pp. 16–18.
179. *Ku-chin T'u-shu Chi-ch'êng*, vol. 432, p. 35.
180. *Ibid.*, p. 56.
181. *Ch'i-kung-liao-fa Chiang-i*, pp. 22–23.
182. Cf. *ibid.*, pp. 19–24.
183. Cf. *ibid.*, p. 34.
184. Cf. *ibid.*, p. 1; cf. Wogralik, *op. cit.*, pp. 88–94.
185. Cf. *Ch'i-kung-liao-fa Chiang-i*, pp. 6–9; Ch'ên T'ao, *op. cit.*, pp. 6–11.
186. Cf. Ch'ên T'ao, *op. cit.*, pp. 6–11; *Ch'i-kung-liao-fa Chiang-i*, pp. 6–9.
187. Cf. *Zdorove* (Health), Moscow, October 1958, no. 4.
188. *Ch'i-kung-liao-fa Chiang-i*, p. 42.
189. *Ibid.*
190. *Ibid.*, p. 43.
191. *Ibid.*, pp. 43–44.
192. *Ibid.*, p. 54.
193. *Ibid.*, p. 55.
194. *Ibid.*
195. *Ibid.*, p. 57.
196. *Ibid.*
197. *Ibid.*, pp. 71–72.
198. Cf. Hsieh Kuan, *op. cit.*, p. 2508; *Chung-hua I-hsüeh Tsa-chih*, February 1954, no. 2, pp. 146–152.
199. Cf. *Chung-i-hsüeh Kai-lun*, p. 552.
200. Cf. Chamfrault, *op. cit.*, vol. I, p. 270.
201. *Chung-i-hsüeh Kai-lun*, pp. 553–554.
202. Cf. *ibid.*, pp. 555–556.
203. *Ibid.*, pp. 553 f.
204. Cf. *Huang-ti Ling-shu*, chaps. 20, 26.
205. Cf. Yüan Guang, *op. cit.*, pp. 20–24.
206. Cf. *Chung-i-hsüeh Kai-lun*, p. 552; *Ch'i-kung-liao-fa Chiang-i*, pp. 57–58; Wogralik-Wjasmenki, *op. cit.*, pp. 95–96.
207. *Ch'i-kung-liao-fa Chiang-i*, p. 58.
208. Cf. Huard-Ming Wong, *op. cit.*, pp. 171–172.
209. Cf. Chen, *op. cit.*, pp. 7–12.
210. Yang Chêng-fu, *op. cit.*, pp. 4–6; Chen, *op. cit.*, pp. 7–12.
211. Cf. Chen, *op. cit.*, pp. 27–28.

216

212. Yang Chêng-fu, *op. cit.*, pp. 4–6, 41–43; Chen, *op. cit.*, pp. 7–8, 169–180.
213. Cf. Chen, *op. cit.*, p. 3; Wogralik-Wjasmenski, *op. cit.*, pp. 88–95.
214. *Ch'i-kung-liao-fa Chiang-i*, p. 59.
215. Cf. *Chên-chiu-hsüeh*, p. 310.
216. Cf. *ibid.*, pp. 310 f.
217. Cf. *ibid.*, pp. 310–314; *Chung-i-hsüeh Kai-lun*, pp. 413–414.
218. Cf. *Chung-hua I-hsüeh Tsa-chih*, 1955, no. 5, pp. 425–429.
219. Cf. Huard-Ming Wong, *op. cit.*, p. 139; Hsieh Kuan, *op. cit.*, pp. 779–780.
220. Cf. Needham, *op. cit.*, vol. II, p. 145.
221. Cf. Gyenes, *op. cit.*, p. 69.
222. Hsieh Kuan, *op. cit.*, p. 2254.
223. Cf. Székely, *op. cit.*, p. 25.
224. Hsieh Kuan, *op. cit.*, p. 88.
225. Cf. Lee T'ao in the *Chinese Medical Journal*, March–April 1956, pp. 177–191; *Chung-hua I-hsüeh Tsa-chih*, February 1954, no. 2, pp. 146–152; Ibragimov-Ibragimova, *op. cit.*, pp. 10–27; Wogralik-Wjasmenski, *op. cit.*, pp. 48–54.
226. Cf. *Li-shih-shang Kan-hsiang Kan-tso-ti Jên*, pp. 97–99.
227. Cf. *ibid.*, pp. 101–104.
228. *Chinese Medical Journal*, 1954, vol. 74, p. 186.
229. *Ibid.*, pp. 186–187.
230. *Ibid.*, p. 185.
231. *Ibid.*, p. 183.
232. *Ibid.*, p. 187.
233. Cf. Ibragimov-Ibragimova, *op. cit.*
234. Cf. *Chung-i-hsüeh Kai-lun*, pp. 233–238.
235. Cf. *ibid.*, pp. 233–318.
236. *Ibid.*, pp. 238–240.
237. *Pên-ts'ao Kang-mu*, vols. I–VI; Chamfrault, *op. cit.*, vol. III· Ibragimov-Ibragimova, *op. cit.*
238. Cf. *Chung-i-hsüeh Kai-lun*, pp. 233–318; *Pên-ts'ao Kang-mu.*
239. Cf. Kérdö, *op. cit.*, pp. 91–102; Bachmann, *op. cit.*, pp. 73–74; Wogralik, *op. cit.*, pp. 38–43; Stiefvater, *Die Organuhr* (Organ Mechanism), Ulm.
240. Cf. *Chung-i-hsüeh Kai-lun*, pp. 233–245.
241. Ibragimov-Ibragimova, *op. cit.*, pp. 279–281.
242. Cf. *Chung-i-hsüeh Kai-lun*, pp. 224–226.
243. Lu Wei-po and Yu Yung-ching, *op. cit.*, p. 33.
244. *Ibid.*
245. *Chinese Medical Journal*, 1957, vol. 75, no. 2, p. 167.
246. *Shih Chi*, chap. 6.
247. A. Waley, *The Poetry and Career of Li-po*, London, 1950, p. 54.
248. Cf. *ibid.*
249. Ibragimov-Ibragimova, *op. cit.*, pp. 186–187.
250. Kuo Mo-jo, *Jugendjahre* (Early Years), Budapest (Europa Publishing House), 1961, pp. 140–146.
251. Ling Yang, *op. cit.*, p. 21.
252. Cf. *Chinese Therapeutical Methods of Acupuncture and Moxibustion*, pp. 1–6.

217

253. Cf. Ling Yang, *op. cit.*, p. 22.
254. Cf. *ibid.*, p. 23
255. Cf. *ibid.*
256. Cf. *ibid.*
257. Cf. Lu Wei-po and Yu Yung-ching, *op. cit.*, p. 33.
258. *Chung-i Tsa-chih*, 1956, vol. 42, no. 2, pp. 114–117.
259. *Ibid.*, pp. 126–128.
260. *Chinese Medical Journal*, 1956, vol. 74, no. 2, p. 202.
261. *Chung-i Tsa-chih*, 1956, vol. 42, no. 2, pp. 167–168.
262. *Chung-hua I-hsüeh Tsa-chih*, 1955, No. 5, pp. 425–428.
263. *Ibid.*, pp. 784–785.
264. Cf. Fedorov, *op. cit.*, pp. 76–77; Wogralik, *op. cit.*, pp. 301–313; Wogralik-Wjasmenski, *op. cit.*, pp. 174–177; Ingamdschanov, *op. cit.*, p. 138.
265. *Renmin Ribao*, November 20, 1958.
266. Cf. *Renmin Ribao*, November 20, 1958; Ling Yang, *op. cit.*, p. 23.
267. Lu Wei-po and Yu Yung-ching, *op. cit.*, p. 32.

BIBLIOGRAPHY

GENERAL SOURCES

ABRÁHAM-BENDE-MEGYERI, *Anatómia-Biológia* (Anatomy and Biology), Budapest (Textbook Press), 1958. —*Chinese Medical Journal*, Chinese Medical Association, Peking. —*Chung-i Ch'ang-yung Ming-tz'û Chien-shih* (Basic Guide to the Commonest Terms Used in Chinese Medicine), Chengtu, Szechuan (National Press), 1959. —*Chung-kuo Ku-tai K'o-hsüeh-chia* (Scholars of Ancient China), Peking (Scientific Literature Press), 1959. —GIOVANNINI-SZATHMÁRI, *Gyógynövényeink* (Medicinal Herbs of Our Native Land), Budapest (Agricultural Literature Press), 1961. GYENES, ISTVÁN, *Nagy orvosi felfedezések* (Important Medical Discoveries), Budapest (Medicina Press), 1961. —HO HUAI-TÊ and TIEN LI-CHÊ, *O-ying-chung I-hsüeh Tz'û-hui* (Russian/English/Chinese Medical Dictionary), Peking (Public Health Press), 1954. —HSIEH KUAN, *Chung-kuo I-hsüeh Ta-tz'û-tien* (Pocket Dictionary of Traditional Chinese Medicine), 4 vols., Shanghai (Commercial Press), 1954. —HUARD, PIERRE, *Structure de la Médecine Chinoise* (Structure of Chinese Medicine), Paris, 1957. —HUARD, PIERRE and MING WONG, *La Médecine Chinoise au cours des siècles,* Paris (Roger Dacosta), 1959 (ET, *Chinese Medicine,* New York [McGraw-Hill], 1968). —IVANOV-SMOLENSKI, *Die Grundzüge der Pathopysiologie der höheren Nerventätigkeit* (The Basic Principles of the Physiopathology of Higher Nervous Activity), Berlin (Academy Press), 1954. —*Ku-chin T'u-shu Chi-ch'êng* (a collection of old and new pictures and books; 18th-century Imperial Encyclopedia), *Encyclopedia I,* new issue in the form of a photolithographic reproduction of the "palace" edition, 800th part, Peking, 1934. —*Ku-chin T'u-shu Chi-ch'êng I-pu Ch'üan-lu* (Medical Works in the Imperial Encyclopedia), *Encyclopedia III,* 12 vols., Peking (Public Health Press), 1962/63. —KUO MO-JO, *Shih*

219

P'i-pan Shu (Book of Tenfold Criticism), Peking (National Press), 1954. —*La-hua I-hsüeh Tzû-tien* (Latin/Chinese Medical Dictionary), Shanghai (Hsinan Medical Press), 1953. —*Li-shih-shang Kan-hsiang Kan-tso-ti Jên* (Men Who Thought and Created in the Course of History), Shanghai (National Press), 1958. —LI T'AO, "The Story of Chinese Medicine," in *China Reconstructs*, September 1955. —LI T'AO, *Chung-kuo I-hsüeh Fa-chan-shih Ta-kang* (A Historical Account of the Development of Chinese Medicine), in *Chung-hua I-hsüeh Tsa-chih*, no. 2, 1954, pp. 146–152. —LING YANG, *Integrating Chinese and Western Medicine*, in *Peking Review*, December 23, 1958. —MAGYARI-PETRÁNYI, *A belgyógyászat alapvonalai* (Basic Principles of Internal Medicine), 2 vols., Budapest (Public Health Press), 1953. —MAO TSO-PÊN, *O-mên Tsu-hsien-ti Ch'uang-tsao Fa-ming* (Ancient Discoveries in Our Country), Shanghai (National Press), 1957. —NEEDHAM, JOSEPH, *Science and Civilisation in China*, Cambridge (Cambridge University Press), I: 1954, II: 1956. —PÁLOS, STEPHAN, *Chung-la I-hsüeh Tzu-hui* (Chinese/Latin Medical Dictionary), manuscript, Budapest, 1962. —PAVLOV, I. P., *Sämtliche Werke* (Collected Works), Berlin (Academy Press), 1953–54. —SAYED INDRIES SHAH, *Oriental Magic*, London (Rider), 1956. —SZÉKELY, SÁNDOR, *Az orvostudomány története* (History of Medicine), Budapest (Medicina Press), 1960. —*T'ai-p'ing Yü Lan* (Encyclopedia of the Emperor Tai Tsung), Encyclopedia II, photolithographic reproduction of the original Sung period edition (Commercial Press), 1935. —WOGRALIK, W. G. and E. S. WJASMENSKI, *Otscherki kitajskogo medizinü* (An Account of Chinese Medicine), Moscow (Medgiz), 1961. —YÜ YÜN-HSIU, *Ku-tai Chi-ping Ming-hou Shu-i* (Interpretation of Old Chinese Names for Illnesses), Peking (Public Health Press), 1955. —YÜAN GUANG, *I Ching* (Book of Changes), Munich-Planegg (Otto Wilhelm Barth Press), 1951.

SPECIAL SOURCES

BACHMANN, G., *Die Akupunktur eine Ordnungstherapie* (Acupuncture as Remedial Therapy), 2 vols., Ulm/Danube (Haug Press), 1959. —CHAMFRAULT, A., *Traité de Médecine Chinoise* (A Treatise on Chinese Medicine), 3 vols., Angoulême (Coquemard Press), I: 1954, II: 1957, III: 1959. —CHANG CHUNG-CHING, *Shang-han Lun Yü Han* (= *Chin Kui Yao Lüeh;* an abridged version of *The*

Golden Shrine), new edition of this work which dates back to the Han period, Peking (National Press), 1955. —CHANG CHUNG-CHING, *Shang-han Lun Yü-i* (Treatise on the Various Kinds of Fevers), new edition with commentary by the Research Institute for Traditional Chinese Medicine, Peking (Public Health Press), 1962. —CHANG WÊN-YÜAN, *T'ai-chi-chüan Ch'ang-shih Wên-t'i Chieh-ta* (Treatise on the General Art of Physiotherapy), Peking (National Callisthenics Press), 1958. —CHEN, YEARNING K., *T'ai-chi Ch'üan, Its Effects and Practical Applications,* Shanghai (Millington), 1947. —*Chên-chiu-hsüeh* (Textbook of Acupuncture and Moxibustion), compiled by the members of the Kiangsu Provincial Academy of Traditional Medicine, Nanking (Kiangsu Provincial Press), 1959. —*Chên-chiu-hsüeh Chiang-i* (Papers on Acupuncture and Moxibustion), edited by the research groups of the Academy of Traditional Medicine in Nanking and Peking, Peking (Public Health Press), 1962. —*Chên-chiu Ju-mên* (An Introduction to Acupuncture and Moxibustion), Peking (Public Health Press), 1959. —CH'EN T'AO, *Ch'i-kung K'e-hsüeh Ch'ang-shih* (General Treatise on Respiratory Therapy), Shanghai (Scientific and Technical Press), 1958. —*Ch'i-kung-liao-fa Chiang-i* (Papers on Respiratory Therapy), edited by the members of the fact-finding group of the Institute for Respiratory Therapy in Shanghai, Shanghai (Scientific and Technical Press), 1958. —*Chien-i Chên-chiu-hsüeh* (A Simple and Easily Understood Summary of Acupuncture and Moxibustion), edited by the East Chinese Medical Academy in Shanghai, Shanghai (Scientific and Technical Press), 1959. —*Chinese Therapeutical Methods of Acupuncture and Moxibustion,* compiled by the Research Institute for Acupuncture and Moxibustion, Peking (Foreign Language Press), 1960. —CHU LIEN, *Hsin Chên-chiu-hsüeh* (Textbook of Modern Acupuncture and Moxibustion), Peking (Public Health Press), 1956. —*Chung-hua I-hsüeh Tsa-chih* (Chinese Medical Journal), Peking (Public Health Press). —*Chung-i-hsüeh Kai-lun* (Summary of Traditional Chinese Medicine), edited by the teaching staff of the Academy of Traditional Medicine in Nanking, Peking (Public Health Press), 1959. —*Chung-i T'ui-na-hsüeh Chiang-i* (Papers on Traditional Chinese Remedial Massage), edited by the Academy of Traditional Medicine in Shanghai, Peking (Public Health Press), 1962. —*Chung-kuo Shou-i-hsüeh Tsa-chih* (Veterinary Science Journal), Peking (Scientific Press). —*Chung-yao-hsüeh Kai-lun* (Summary of Chinese Pharmacology), edited by the Academies of Traditional Chinese Medicine in Nanking and Peking, Peking (Public Health Press), 1959. —DSCHANG HUI-

DJIÄN, *Li Schidschen, der grosse chinesische Pharmakologe des 16. Jahrhunderts* (Li Shih-chên, the great 16th-Century Chinese Pharmacologist), Peking, 1959. —FEDOROV, I. I., *Otscherki po narodnoj kitajskoi medizine* (Treatise on Chinese Folk Medicine), Moscow (Medgiz Press), 1960. —*Hsi-i Hsüeh-hsi Chung-i Lun-wên Hsüan-chi* (Western Medicine Acquires Traditional Methods—Collected Articles), edited by the Research Institute of Traditional Medicine, vol. I, Peking (Public Health Press), 1959. —HUANG CHIA-SSU, in *China Reconstructs,* June 1960. —*Huang-ti Ling-shu* (the "Ling Shu" section of *The Yellow Emperor's Classic of Internal Medicine*), in *Encyclopedia I:* nos. 428–430; in *Encyclopedia III:* vol. II, *Huang-ti Nei-ching Su-wên I-shih* (*The Yellow Emperor's Classic of Internal Medicine* Translated into Modern Chinese), edited by the teaching staff of the Academy of Traditional Chinese Medicine in Nanking, Shanghai (Scientific and Technical Press), 1959. —*Huang-ti Su-wên* (the "Su Wên" section of *The Yellow Emperor's Classic of Internal Medicine*), in *Encyclopedia I:* vol. I, *I-tsung Chin-chien* (*The Golden Mirror of the Art of Healing*), 1749. —IBRAGIMOV, F. and W. IBRAGIMOVA, *Osnovnüe lekarstvenüe sredstva kitajskoi medizinü* (The Basic Medicaments Used in Chinese Medicine), Moscow (Medgiz Press), 1960. —INGAMD-SCHANOV, N. I., *Praktitscheskoe rukovodstvo po igloterapii* (Practical Handbook of Acupuncture), Tashkent (Medgiz Press), 1960. —KÉRDÖ, ISTVAN, *Idöjárás, éghajlat, egészség* (Weather, Climate and Health), Budapest (Medicina Press), 1961. —LEE T'AO, *Achievements in Materia Medica During the Ming Dynasty* (*1368–1643*), in *Chinese Medical Journal,* no. 74, 1956. —LI SHIH-CHÊN, *Pên-ts'ao Kang-mu* (Book of Medicaments), reprint of a book which first appeared in the Ming period, Shanghai (Commercial Press), 1954. —LIU KUI-CHÊN, *Ch'i-kung-liao-fa Shih-chien* (Practical Application of Chinese Respiratory Therapy), Paoting (Hopei Provincial Press), 1957. —LU CHIH-CHÜN, *Hsin-pien Chên-chiu-hsüeh* (Modern Handbook of Acupuncture and Moxibustion), Chungking (Chungking National Press), 1958. —LU WEI-PO and YU YUNG-CHING, *Learning from Ancient China's Medicine* in *China Reconstructs,* October 1959. —MANAKA, YOSHIO and H. SCHMIDT, *Chên-shu-ti Chin-tai Yen-chiu* (Modern Research into Acupuncture), Chinese translation, Peking (Public Health Press), 1958. —MASPERO, HENRI, *Les procédés de nourrir le principe vital dans la réligion taoiste ancienne,* in the *Journal Asiatique,* 1937, pp. 182, 197, 380, 409–411. —*Nan Ching* (Book of Ailments), in *Encyclopedia I,* no. 430. —*Shanghai Zhong-yi-yao Zazhi* (Shanghai

222

Journal of Chinese Medicine and Pharmacology), Traditional Medical Society, Shanghai. —SOULIÉ DE MORANT, *Précis de la vraie acupuncture chinoise,* Paris (Mercure de France), 1955. —STIEFVATER, E. W., *Was ist Akupunktur? Wie wirkt Akupunktur?* (What Is Acupuncture? How Does Acupuncture Work?), Ulm/Danube (Haug Press), 1955. —STIEFVATER, E. W., *Akupunktur als Neuraltherapie* (Acupuncture as Neurotherapy), Ulm/Danube (Haug Press), 1956. —*T'ai-chi-ch'üan Yün-tung* (Therapeutic Exercises), 3 vols., Peking (National Callisthenics Press), 1958. —Ts'AO HSI-CHEN, *Wai-shang Chung-i An-mo-liao-fa* (Traditional Methods of Massage in Rehabilitation), Peking (National Callisthenics Press), 1962. —WANG HSÜEH-TAI, *Chên-chiu-hsüeh Shou-ts'e* (Handbook of Acupuncture and Moxibustion), Peking (Public Health Press), 1959. —WANG SHU-HE, *Mai Ching* (Book of the Pulse), in *Encyclopedia I:* no. 430. —WOGRALIK, W. G., *Osnovü kitajskogo letschebnogo metoda tschen-ziu* (Basic Principles of the Chinese Therapeutic Methods of Acupuncture and Moxibustion), Gorki (Gorki Press), 1961. —YANG CHENG-FU, *T'ai-chi-ch'üan T'i-yung Ch'üan-shu* (Remedial Therapy Library), Peking (National Callisthenics Press), 1957. —YANG CHI-CHOU, *Chên-chiu Ta-ch'êng (Compendium of Acupuncture and Moxibustion)*, reprint of the book which first appeared during the Ming period, Peking (Public Health Press), 1962. —*Yao-hsüeh Hsüeh-pao* (Pharmacological Journal), Chinese Academy of Science, Peking.

INDEX OF NAMES

224

225

INDEX OF SUBJECTS

226

227

231

232

234

235